Therapeutic Humor
with the Elderly

Therapeutic Humor with the Elderly

Francis A. McGuire
Rosangela K. Boyd
Ann James

The Haworth Press, Inc.
New York • London • Norwood (Australia)

Therapeutic Humor with the Elderly has also been published as *Activities, Adaptation & Aging*, Volume 17, Number 1 1992.

The Haworth Press, Inc., 10 Alice Street, Binghamton, NY 13904-1580 USA

Library of Congress Cataloging-in-Publication Data

Therapeutic humor with the elderly / Francis A. McGuire, Rosangela K. Boyd, Ann James.
     p. cm.
     Includes bibliographical references.
     ISBN 1-56024-310-4 (acid-free paper)
     1. Wit and humor–Therapeutic use. 2 Aged–Rehabilitation. 3. Nursing home care. 4. Wit and humor in medicine. I. McGuire, Francis A. II. Boyd, Rosangela K. III. James, Ann.
RC953.8.H85M38 1993
615.8'51–dc20   92-43465
                                                 CIP

Therapeutic Humor with the Elderly

CONTENTS

ABOUT THE AUTHORS

Francis A. McGuire, PhD, is Professor of Therapeutic Recreation in the Department of Parks, Recreation, and Tourism Management at Clemson University. He is an active teacher and researcher in the field of gerontology and has published in a variety of journals. Dr. McGuire has presented papers and workshops at national, regional, state, and local conferences on topics such as patterns of outdoor recreation participation by older individuals, the role of humor in long term care facilities, and constraints to leisure involvement in retirement.

Rosangela K. Boyd, PhD, is Assistant Professor in the Department of Sports Management and Leisure Studies at Temple University. A certified therapeutic recreation specialist, she is familiar with the realities of long term care. In addition to therapeutic humor, Dr. Boyd is interested in the areas of choice and control, developmental disabilities, and cultural diversity as they relate to older adults. She has contributed to the professional literature on gerontology and has given presentations at various conferences and workshops for activity directors.

Ann James, PhD, Associate Professor in the Department of Parks, Recreation, and Tourism Management at Clemson University, speaks widely on the therapeutic applications of humor. She has experience as a recreation therapist in general medical and mental health facilities and has served as a consultant to long term care facilities. Dr. James was a member of the Board of Directors of the American Therapeutic Recreation Association and President of the National Therapeutic Recreation Society.

Foreword

We have all heard that laughter is the best medicine and probably have not thought a great deal about it. The claim has never been tested by the FDA, has never resulted in the expenditure of millions of research dollars designed to test its accuracy and has never caused a congressional investigation. In fact, it resides in the same, largely untested, world as "absence makes the heart grow fonder" and "out of sight, out of mind." This book examines the role of humor in the therapeutic process. It is not the first book to do so and will not be the last. However, it is unique in its focus on long term care facilities. It is designed to provide an overview of what is currently known about the role of humor in therapy as well as to provide specific suggestions which will be helpful in incorporating humor into the activity program in long term care facilities. The role of the AARP Andrus Foundation in providing funding for the Clemson Humor Project was a major impetus for this work. We gratefully acknowledge their support. In addition, we are indebted to Bettye Cecil and the White Oak Manor Corporation.

Chapter I

Introduction

Most of us are aware of the graying of America. Average life expectancy has increased and a person reaching sixty-five years of age can expect to live an additional 16.9 years (AARP, 1989). More people are living longer than ever before. Clearly the quantity of life has increased. An issue for activity professionals is how to assist in the enhancement of the quality of life as well. The challenge of increasing the quality of life may be particularly difficult for residents of long term care facilities.

In 1985, 1.3 million persons aged 65 or older lived in long term care facilities. Although this figure represents no more than 5% of the population, percentages increase dramatically with age. While approximately 1% of persons aged 65-74 live in nursing homes, the percentage increases to 6% for those 75-84 years old and 22% for those 85 years of age or older (AARP, 1989). Since the 85 and over age group reflects one of the fastest growing minorities in America, it can be expected that the nursing home population will increase in the future. As a result, meeting the needs of this group will become increasingly important.

THE QUALITY OF LIFE IN LONG TERM CARE FACILITIES

George and Bearon (1980) define quality of life in terms of four underlying dimensions: two objective and two subjective. The objective dimensions are general health/functional status and socioeconomic status. The subjective dimensions are life satisfaction and self-esteem. One of the concerns of activity professionals is with improving the quality of life, particularly its subjective components, for the residents of long term care facilities. Recreation has the potential to benefit residents in a variety of ways which directly impact quality of life. However, carefully designed programs based on knowledge of the benefits of activities are required.

The transition from one's home to a long term care facility can be a very difficult one. Loss of social groups, loss of possessions, loss of privacy, loss of physical space, loss of mobility, loss of independence and loss of control are unfortunate concomitants of relocation into a long term care facility. Residents may develop feelings of helplessness as a result of loss of control (Langer & Rodin, 1976; Mercer & Kane, 1979; Abramson, Garber & Seligman, 1980; Langer, 1983; Voelkl, 1986; Baltes & Baltes, 1986). Measures to help individuals maintain control, develop coping skills and develop a positive attitude toward life are necessary. Activity personnel are often at the forefront of this effort.

Kelly (undated) states that continuity "is associated with resources that enable those whose abilities and social circles are being reduced, to stay engaged, to act in ways to continue to express what they are and what they intend to be." When those resources are present, individuals are able to maintain dignity and autonomy, thus being more likely to regard life positively and retain favorable views of themselves. The opportunity to preserve identity and skill, then, impacts on the subjective dimensions of the quality of life mentioned earlier.

Activities can play an important role in preserving feelings of effectiveness as well as assisting in adjustment to the long term care environment through the provision of opportunities for engagement and continuity (Havighurst, 1972). Through involvement in recreation activity, independence, control, growth and variety can be incorporated into the daily lives of residents.

Stimulation and variety in activities are important in retaining interest and motivation among many residents. It has been found that the less stimulation one receives, the less resistant to external pressures one becomes (Namehow & Lawton, 1976). It has been suggested that individuals prefer to become involved in arousing experiences, opting for variety rather than optimality (Walt, 1978; Duellman, Barris & Kielhofner, 1986). Stimulation can be introduced by the implementation of innovative programs that capture the interest and stimulate the mind of individuals. One type of intervention that may bring new life into the nursing home setting, be a force in improving the quality of life, and provide continuity to life, is humor.

THE POTENTIAL ROLE OF HUMOR IN THERAPY

Laughter is a daily occurrence and universal experience. We have all laughed and have all made other people laugh. Humor is often used in the performance of job related duties. Humor is utilized in the reduction of stress. A number of books have been written about humor and laughter. Some have been academic in their approach (see, for example, Chapman & Foot, 1977; Morreall, 1983; McGhee & Goldstein, 1983). Others are more "self-help" types of books designed to assist the reader in using humor in life (Blumenfield & Alpern, 1986; Peter & Dana, 1982; Klein, 1989). Nevertheless the role of humor as part of a therapeutic process requires further empirical examination.

If the benefits of humor could be packaged and sold in pill-form, the rush to pharmacies would be tremendous. A variety of authors (Klein, 1989; Cousins, 1979; Robinson, 1983 McGhee & Goldstein book; Salameh, 1983; Haig, 1988) have identified the benefits of humor and laughter.

A recent publication (Ewers, Jacobson, Powers & McConney, 1983) noted that "the effect of humor on physical and mental health has been long noted." In addition, the belief that laughter is the best medicine is part of our culture. Although that may be the case, it has not been well documented in the literature. There is anecdotal support for such a position. (See, for example, Cousins, 1979.) However, few systematic attempts have been made to verify, through rigorous research designs, the importance of laughter in physical and mental health. Much of the literature that exists is in the field of psychotherapy and limited in its applicability to activity programs in long term care facilities.

Although humor is commonly believed to possess therapeutic value, more scientific investigation is needed to confirm this belief. Examination of the therapeutic properties of humor was greatly stimulated by the awareness of Norman Cousins' story. Suffering from ankylosing spondylitis, Cousins received little encouragement from his doctors. Taking responsibility for his own care, he chose to "cure" himself through large doses of vitamin C and laughter. Cousins (1979) not only reported requiring less pain medication and being better able to fall asleep following regular sessions of hearty laughter, but his sedimentation rate also decreased over time. Eventually the inflammation in his joints subsided and he was declared cured. Although not absolutely sure laughter was the primary agent of his cure, Cousins suggested his improvement resulted from a relationship between a positive frame of mind and successful health outcomes. His hypothesis was that if negative emotions are detrimental to health, positive emotions may have the reverse effect. Cousins' story provides ample opportunity for speculating about the therapeutic efficacy of humor.

Recently, increasing research efforts have been geared toward the empirical examination of humor and therapy. Research findings, to be discussed in detail in Chapter II, indicate that humor has the potential to produce positive effects in the cardiopulmonary and musculoskeletal systems of the body (Fry, 1986). Humor has also been shown to reduce anxiety (Nemeth, 1979), increase morale (Simon, 1988), and mediate the relationship between stress and mood disturbance (Martin & Lefcourt, 1983).

Levine (1977) indicated laughter can relieve anxiety, develop ego mastery, and provide a message that everything is all right. He went on to state that humor enables individuals to face their fears, whether they originate from internal or external sources. If Levine's perspective is an accurate one, laughter can be a major tool in developing positive feelings in residents of long term care facilities. These individuals may require affirmation of their importance, reduction in stress and anxiety, and some sense of normalcy. In fact, Kahana, Liang and Felton (1980) found that environmental stimulation is an effective tool in improving the quality of life for residents of long term care facilities. Humor is one way to introduce stimulation into long term care facilities. It is a link with the past and an affirmation of continuing life and vitality. It may have a major impact on the lives of individuals in long term care facilities.

Residing in a long term care facility requires the ability to adjust and cope. Humor has been shown to be an effective tool in coping with stress (Robinson, 1977; Martin & Lefcourt, 1983; Namehow, 1986). When this finding is viewed in conjunction with the documented relationship between humor and maturity as well as successful adjustment (Grotjahn, 1957; O'Connel, 1960; Anthony & Benedik, 1975; Namehow, 1986), it is likely that the introduction of humor into long term care facilities will produce positive effects related to the quality of residents' lives.

Simon (1988) indicated that a sense of well-being is dependent on the individual's ability to perceive his or her current situation with its limitations and focus his or her energy on development and growth. Such an approach requires a positive outlook on life. Humor may be one tool in developing such a positive outlook, even in the presence of unpleasant realities such as disability and loss. Robinson (1977) stated that humor is "first and foremost an attitude towards life; a willingness to accept life and accept ourselves with a shrug and a smile, with a certain lightheartedness . . . this is not a sense of resignation or indifference, but rather a sense of mastery over life" (p. 134).

Humor has also been viewed as a way of looking at a situation from a different point of view, diffusing a crisis and providing an opportunity for increased insight and objectivity (Crane, 1990). Sullivan and Deane (1988) supported this perspective on humor. They wrote "humor allows the person to defuse anger and/or frustration associated with a distressful event by focusing on its comical elements" (p. 20). Chapter IV will discuss ways to incorporate humor into situations and events experienced throughout life, even those which may appear to be without much humor. The activities provided in that chapter will facilitate development of a humor rich environment which may counteract the frustrations and anger experienced by residents of long term care facilities.

The ability of humor to generate pleasure (Levine, 1977) points toward its potential role in bringing about positive affect in residents of long term care facilities. Residents of long term care facilities may experience little emotion as a result of a lack of stimulation and variety in the facility. Humor may be an effective weapon in counteracting this phenomenon. In fact, there is evidence that humor is positively correlated with elevation in mood and morale in institutionalized older adults (Ewers, Jacobson, Powers & McConney, 1983; Napora, 1984; Simon, 1988).

Not only is humor effective in bringing about positive psycho-social changes in residents of long term care facilities, it may also be an effective tool in facilitating physical changes. Among the most debilitating aspects of aging is the occurrence of frequent and persistent pain. Pain interferes with activities of daily living and may negatively influence mental health as a result of increased dependence and decreased ability to experience pleasure. There is a need for interventions which will decrease the pain experienced by older individuals. Cousins (1979) believed laughter was the enemy of pain. Peter and Dana (1982) suggested humor can control pain in four ways: distraction, relaxation, attitude, and hormonal activity. The development of a humor program may, therefore, provide relief from debilitating pain for residents of long term care facilities.

One of the only attempts to examine the role humor can play in long term care facilities was part of a program conducted by the Andrus Volunteers of the Ethel Percy Andrus Gerontology Center at the University of Southern California (Ewers, Jacobson, Powers & McConney, 1983). It was a comprehensive program which incorporated a variety of approaches to introduce humor into a nursing home environment. The intent of the project at its inception was to develop and evaluate the effects of a humor program on residents of long term care facilities. Although a variety of methodological difficulties precluded scientific evaluation of the program, observations of residents provided insight into the benefits of the program. Over 60 residents participated in the program. (See Chapter II for a complete description of this program.) Observed changes in the participants included: increased awareness of others; appreciation for the program; anticipation of the program; enjoyment of discussion of previous programs; more outgoing, positive attitudes; increased socialization; increased likelihood of using humor in interactions with others; increased enjoyment; and increased initiative. As the author of the report concluded: ''the project must be seen as a success on the basis of the effectiveness of the Humor Program in altering the behavior patterns and expectations of the residents'' (p. 60).

A study by Adams and McGuire (1986) provided additional support for the use of humor in long term care facilities. (See Chapter II for a complete description of this research.) They found evidence that humor may be effective in reducing pain and increasing affect in residents of long term care facilities. These two projects point toward the potential benefits of using humor in long term care facilities. However, more efforts are needed to establish this link. This collection is designed to do that.

WHAT'S TO COME

The remainder of this volume is divided into three chapters.The next chapter provides an overview of humor and its role in therapy. A growing body of literature related to humor is developing. Some is research based and some is anecdotal. All of it is useful. This section will provide an overview of this literature. In addition, an overview of theoretical conceptualizations of humor will be included.

Chapter III of this publication is a report on the Clemson Humor Project. This year long study examined the efficacy of humor in improving the quality of life for residents of long term care facilities. It is one of the few experimental or quasi-experimental studies designed to determine the therapeutic efficacy of humor. In addition, it is one of the few empirical examinations of humor in long term care facilities. The results clearly indicated the potential value of humor in nursing homes.

It is our belief that humor programs can be developed in any facility. There is no need to be able to tell jokes or funny stories to incorporate humor into a program. Humor is all around us in every day events, in the newspaper, in our friends. The effective use of humor requires the ability to find it. The fourth section of this work will help do that. It provides techniques for incorporating humor into the activity program.

Chapter II

Theoretical and Research Perspectives on Humor

The trajectory of humor in history resembles that of leisure and play. In fact, the concepts of humor and play have been linked by a number of authors (Levine, 1970, Mindess, 1977; Fry & Allen, 1976; McGhee, 1979; Fry, 1982; Mannel & MacMahon, 1982). Mannel and McMahon (1982) posited that humor is "one form of play that appears to accompany many non-leisure activities while also being the basis of some forms of entertainment that engage people during leisure" (p. 143).

Both humor and play have received much criticism in the past, especially during years of religious repression and extreme valuation of work. As society evolved and new values emerged, the importance of humor and other forms of play began to be recognized as beneficial to psychological well-being. In fact, recent efforts have focused on using these benefits as part of the therapeutic process for individuals with special needs.

THEORETICAL PERSPECTIVES

Although it is not the purpose of this manuscript to provide a major treatise on the theories explaining humor, some insight into the underlying dynamics of humor is helpful in developing a humor program. Understanding factors which foster humor will provide an approach to creating humor.

Although there has been interest by theoreticians in determining what makes a particular stimulus appreciated as humorous and in the responses to the presentation of such stimuli, most theories focus on the process mediating the exposure to the stimulus and the reaction to it. The most popular theories of humor can be classified as either cognitive, psychosocial or physiological.

Cognitive Theories

The incongruity theory has received a great deal of attention by researchers interested in the cognitive process associated with the production and appreciation of humor. The theory postulates that laughter is "an intellectual reaction to something unexpected, illogical or inappropriate" (Williams, 1986, p. 14). Supposedly, the world is organized in an orderly pattern known and shared by most people. When the pattern is broken, creating a gap between what one expects and what actually happens, then incongruity results.

Advocates of such a framework appeared in the 18th and 19th centuries. One of the most famous, Kant (1892), proposed that "in everything that is to excite a lively convulsive laughter, there must be something absurd. Laughter is an affection arising from the transformation of a strained expectation into nothing" (p. 223). Schopenhauer (1964) expanded Kant's version by claiming that his predecessor's use of "nothing" did not accurately describe the mechanism of incongruity. Rather, he believed that instead of the normal anticipated result, people perceived something that clashed with their expectations.

Because of their pure cognitive nature, incongruity theories do not address psychosocial traits of the humor experience. Therefore, a further approach to understanding humor is needed.

Psychosocial Theories

Two major categories of theories can be described as psychosocial theories. They are classified as superiority and relief theories.

Superiority theory. The concept of superiority in explaining humor can be traced back to the Greek philosophers. Aristotle saw laughter as a form of derision. To him, the laughable person was one who perceived himself as "wealthier, better looking, more virtuous or wiser" than he really was (Morreal, 1983, p. 5).

Superiority theories deal with hostility and aggression. They call attention to the fact that enjoyment is often derived from exposing weakness and deformities of others, putting down individuals or groups (Zillmann, 1983). Hobbes (1840) recognized as the first proponent of a superiority theory, defined laughter as " a sudden glory arising from some conception of some eminency in ourselves, by comparison with the infirmity of others, or with our own formerly" (McGhee, 1979, p. 5).

Anthropologic studies point to the inherently aggressive nature of laughter (Lorenz, 1966). It is seen as an evolutionary mechanism by which the individual expresses a feeling of greater adaptation to his enemy (Ludovici, 1933). Rapp (1951) interpreted laughter as originating from one primitive behavior, "the war of triumph in an ancient jungle duel" (p. 43-44). Although combat is no longer a fact of daily life today, people still laugh at mistakes and misfortunes of others. Rapp (1951) does admit to a more benevolent attitude toward the person being laughed at in modern society, although the feeling of superiority is still present. Martineau (1972) perceptively noted that the sense of superiority producing mirth results only from derision of objects with whom the individual does not identify. A typical illustration of this proposition is the negative reaction by members of a certain minority group to jokes disparaging their own group.

Although it is undeniable that certain humorous situations result from the emotions associated with superiority, not all humorous experiences must have elements of disparagement. Not all humor is a result of social confrontation; other elements such as tension relief can account for humor and laughter.

Relief theories. Although psychosocial theories have a physiological component–venting of energy–they also have a strong psychological component since it is "nervous" energy that is released with humor. According to McGhee (1979) there are two ways in which laughter can bring about relief. "The person may have come into the situation with the nervous energy that is to be released or the laughter situation itself may cause the build up of the nervous energy, as well as its release" (p. 21). Traditional social prohibitions, such as those related to sex and violence, can lead to pent-up nervous energy that is released by laughter when someone breaks the taboo and talks about them.

Spencer's position was that when feelings regarded as inappropriate build up, the release of energy is obtained by laughter. Dewey (1894) similarly stated that laughter was a "sudden relaxation of strain, so far as occurring through the medium of breathing and the vocal apparatus" (p. 559).

In his paper "Humour," Freud (1959) talked about the grandeur and elevation associated with humor.

> He stated: "The grandeur in it clearly lies in the triumph of narcissism, the victorious assertion of the ego's invulnerability. The ego refuses to be distressed by the provocations of reality, to let itself be compelled to suffer. It insists that it cannot be affected by the traumas of the external world; it shows, in fact, that such traumas are no more than occasions for it to gain pleasure." (p. 162)

Thoughts and feelings that society forces us to suppress can be let into our conscious minds by the use of jokes. To Freud, jokes allowed individuals to "waive restrictions and open sources of pleasure that have become inaccessible" (p. 147).

Relief theories are another way to explain humor, but do not account for its complexity. One of the criticisms of them is the fact that not all humorous experiences result from unconscious conflicts and liberation of psychic energy.

Physiological Theories

Contrary to the theories discussed above, pure physiological theories are not concerned with explaining the reasons behind mirth and laughter. They attempt to describe the organic process associated with humor.

Berlyne's (1972) incongruity-arousal theory was developed as a reaction to old relief theories. He theorized a two part activation of the human organism during exposure to humorous stimuli. During the arousal phase, there is an increase of nervous system activity. For the process to be completed, a relaxation phase is needed, in which arousal tension is reduced through the resolution of incongruity. As a consequence of the interest aroused by Berlyne's theory, a number of studies were developed to investigate the physiological correlates of humor.

An integration of theories is needed for a comprehensive look at humor. To focus on one and disregard the other is to ignore the enormous complexity of humor, its diverse facets. However, that is beyond the focus of this manuscript. Interested readers are referred to any of several books in this area (for example, Morreal, 1983).

RESEARCH PERSPECTIVES

Humor is regarded as an evolutionary component of human beings. It is manifested in early stages of development; presumably inherited, it is shaped as the individual matures and interacts with his or her environment (McGhee, 1979). To Freud, humor could be viewed as the essence of a mature personality (O' Connel, 1964). Levine (1956) agrees: "It follows that an inability to appreciate humor or deviant responses to it can be regarded as a sensitive indicator of maladjustment and inner disturbances" (p. 35). O'Connel (1960) tested this assumption and found that humor appreciation was indeed observed more frequently among mature, better adjusted persons. Mindess and Turek (1979) sum up the role humor plays during the developmental stages by saying:

> In its earlier stages, our sense of humor frees us from the chains of our perpetual, conventional, logical linguistic, and moral systems. The unexpected act, the startling remark, the nonsense quip, the pun, and the dirty joke are all, in the beginning, parties to our conspiracy to escape. In its more sophisticated stages, it releases us from our naive belief that man is a reasonable, trustworthy creature. . . . To attain its ultimate, however, it must liberate us from identification with our egos, for in this feat resides its quintessential power. (p. 2)

Simon (1988) writes: "the adult's sense of 'success' or well-being, therefore, is dependent significantly on his ability to perceive his current situation with all its limitations and channel energy for development and growth" (p. 11). To fight the unpleasant realities of old age, such as disability, losses and approaching death, one must keep a positive attitude toward life.

Humor has also been interpreted as a way of looking at a situation from a different point of view, lightening up crisis and providing people with an opportunity for increased insight and objectivity (Crane, 1990). "Humor allows the person to defuse anger and/or frustration associated with a distressful event by focusing on its comical elements" (Sullivan & Deane, 1988, p. 20).

Examination of the therapeutic properties of humor have been greatly stimulated by the awareness raised by the Norman Cousins' story. Suffering from a painful and debilitating disease called ankylosing spondylitis, Cousins received little encouragement from his doctors. Taking his health care into his hands, Cousins chose to cure himself through large doses of vitamin C and laughter. According to Cousins (1979), not only did he require less pain medication and was able to sleep better following exposure to regular sessions of hearty laughter, but his sedimentation rate also decreased over time. Eventually, the inflammation in his joints subsided and he was declared cured.

Although not absolutely sure that laughter was the primary and direct agent of cure, Cousins suggested a relationship between a positive frame of mind and successful health outcomes. His hypothesis was that if negative emotions are believed to be detrimental to our health, positive emotions might well have the reverse effect. In Cousins' story, there is room for speculation regarding the physiological and psychological benefits of humor.

Lately, more research has been conducted, not only in the area of physical health, but also on the relationship between humor and indicators of psychological well-being. Research findings indicate that humor has the potential to produce positive effects on the cardiopulmonary and musculoskelatal systems of the body (Fry, 1986). Humor has also been shown to reduce anxiety (Nemeth, 1979), increase morale (Simon, 1988), and mediate the relationship between stress and mood disturbance (Martin & Lefcourt, 1983).

Is Laughter the Best Medicine?

One of the biggest concerns associated with growing old is decline in health (Cumming & Henry, 1961). An undeniable reality of aging is that physical deterioration occurs, although gradually and differently for each individual. While old age brings gains such as wisdom and experience, it also takes away valued abilities related to health, such as energy level, mobility and self care.

While self-perceived good health has been positively correlated with well-being (Lawton 1983), self perceived poor health is associated with decreased happiness and lower activity levels. Beck and Page (1988) found that health was a very important mediator in the relationship between affect and type and levels of activities in which the elderly participate. The ability to engage in activities was found to be more meaningful for those retired men in poor health than for those in good health, yielding significant positive changes in affect.

Lifestyles have to be adjusted to make up for changes in health. As Christensen (1978) has indicated, one's attitude about physical health is an important factor in determining how life is experienced. Chronic conditions such as arthritis and hypertension can cause minor disruptions in lifestyle or become the central determinant of how one chooses to live.

Objective facts are balanced by subjective reality, that is, the way the older person chooses to perceive the situation. As pointed out by Kalish (1977) "when people feel depressed, angry at themselves, or helpless and hopeless, they are more likely to perform overtly self-destructive acts" (p. 159). Many health care professionals believe that psychological orientation affects the body, if not directly, through the behavior that follows from it.

Life stresses have been found to affect health negatively while positive life events have been found to be directly correlated to good self-reported physical health (Weinberger, Darnell, Martz, Hiner, Neill & Tierney, 1986). The correlation between stress and illness, however, is not high, only .30 (Lefcourt & Martin, 1986). Other factors have been suggested to moderate such relationship. Among them, humor has recently been receiving increased attention. Fry, a renowned researcher in the field of physiology and humor, states:

> Stress is antagonized by humor in both its mental and emotional aspect and in its physical aspect. Emotional tension, contributing to stress, is lowered through the cathartic effects

of humor. Mirthful laughter is followed by a state of compensatory physical relaxation, diminishing physical tension. (1979, p. 1)

Because of the positive frame of mind associated with exposure to humor, it is quite possible that by creating opportunities for mirth and laughter, health care professionals may also impact perception of physical heath and possibly, as Cousins suggested (1979), help fight disease. Evidence is accumulating which supports this hypothesis.

Physiological Benefits of Humor

For years, humor has been regarded as naturally good for the mind. Research studies into its physiological benefits did not begin to accumulate until the second half of this century. Below are some of the areas investigated in which humor has been found to have a positive effect.

Musculoskeletal effects. With laughter, skeletal muscles are activated. The activity may be mild or extreme, depending on the intensity of the humor response. Face, scalp, neck, shoulders and even thoracic and abdominal muscles are among those often stimulated. If the response is extreme, muscles of the entire body–like those in arms and legs–may become involved (Fry, 1986).

For the elderly, the muscle stimulation is especially beneficial since those individuals in most need of exercise may be precisely those bound to wheelchairs or beds, thus incapable of participating in other activity modalities.

Muscles not involved in laughter relax (Paskind, 1932; Schwartz, 1974) and after laughter subsides, even those participating muscles relax (Sveback, 1975; Chapman, 1976). This relaxation is significant to the older individual since it is capable of breaking the spasm-pain-spasm cycle that accompanies so many chronic illnesses in old age, such as rheumatism, arthritis and neuralgias.

Cardiac and circulatory effects. Not only is the cardiac muscle stimulated with mirth, but also heart rate and blood pressure accompany the laughter episode (Averill, 1969; Fry & Roder, 1969; Langevin & Day, 1972; Stroufe & Waters, 1976). Following stimulation, both heart rate and blood pressure drop in relation to pre-laughter baseline rates (Scheff & Scheele, 1979; Fry & Savin, 1982). This is significant since studies have shown that regular cardiac exercise decreases the vulnerability for coronary heart disease and speeds rehabilitation from heart attack (Fry, 1986).

For the elderly, heart attacks are the leading cause of death. For sedentary adults, many not exercising the upper extremities of their bodies voluntarily, exposure to laughter episodes may lower the risk of heart attacks (Williams, 1986).

Circulation is also improved during mirth as a result of cardiac stimulation. This may help the older organism fight the formation of blood clots and speed up the movement of oxygen to the tissues and of immune elements, thus helping fight pathology in the elderly (Fry, 1986).

Respiratory effects. The lungs are intensely involved in several mirth responses such as laughing, chuckling and guffawing. Normally, the individual experiences a cyclic breathing pattern, which leaves behind in the lung residual air while absorbing environmental air. As oxygen is removed from residual air to fulfill metabolic demands of the body, residual air develops a build-up of carbon-dioxide and water vapor–metabolic waste products. Such products, when in excess, may favor the growth of bacteria and pulmonary infection (Fry, 1986).

With laughter, cyclic breathing is interrupted, pulmonary ventilation is expanded and secretion in the lungs is expectorated, preventing infection. Fry and Roder (1977) demonstrated the disruption in the respiratory cycle caused by mirthful laughter. Similarly, Fry and Stoft (1971) showed that levels of oxygen in the peripheral blood are maintained during prolonged heavy laughter. With many elderly suffering from respiratory illnesses such as bronchitis, asthma and emphysema, the benefits of humor respiration is clear.

Hormonal effects. From analyzing venous blood samples, collected during exposure to humorous stimuli, Fry, Berk and Tan (Fry, 1986) reported that catecholamine activation can be intense during exposure to humor and laughter. Catecholamines are complex substances associated with alertness. Alertness levels in the elderly are known to gradually decrease, affecting memory and retention. The possibility of enhancing alertness and stimulating memory is certainly an exciting potential of humorous activity. The stimulating effects of humor on memory and alertness were investigated by several researchers using performance on scholastic tests as the dependent variable (Browning, 1979; Ziv, 1982; Young, 1982; McGhee, 1986; Goodman, 1982). Results pointed to the effectiveness of humor in enhancing mental functioning in areas such as learning, creative thinking and memory.

Another possible benefit of humor that has been investigated relates to its anti-inflammatory effect through increased levels of catecholamines in the blood stream (Schacter & Wheeler, 1962). Considering painful inflammatory conditions experienced by the elderly, such as gout and arthritis, evidence of such relationship would be quite welcome.

A recent study by Cogan, Cogan, Waltz and McCue (1987) has generated exciting conclusions regarding the effectiveness of laughter in raising discomfort thresholds. In their first experiment, the researchers measured pressure induced discomfort in 40 subjects who had listened to either laughter inducing, relaxation inducing, dull narrative audio tapes, or no tapes at all. Discomfort thresholds were found to be higher among those listening to both laughter and relaxation tapes. In the second experiment, discomfort was measured in subjects matched for pressure induced discomfort thresholds. After exposure to the stimuli, subjects in the laughter group were found to exhibit higher discomfort thresholds than subjects in any other group. Such results suggest that humor, beyond simple distraction, reduces discomfort sensitivity and thus may be potentially useful as an intervention strategy in the reduction of clinical pain.

A study by Tennant (1986) offered some clinical support for the physiological benefits of humor. The purpose of the study was to determine the effect of humor on the recovery rate of elderly patients following cataract surgery. The sample included twelve women and eight men, ages ranging from 65 to 95 years. All subjects had undergone cataract surgery 24 hours prior to participation in the study. The instrumentation consisted of a short version of the Humor Survey (15 jokes) and questions regarding demographics, background and social data. Patients were approached in their hospital rooms and instructed to answer the questions and proceed to the jokes, rating them from "not at all funny"(1) to "very funny"(4).

Results indicated that there was a positive relationship between recovery rates and humor scores for males, with those scoring the highest in the Humor Survey also having the fastest recovery rates as determined by hospital stay.

More studies and larger samples are necessary in order to generalize findings favoring the use of humor to achieve physiological benefits such as recovery from illness. It is also important that research determines whether recovery is a result of physiological properties of humor or if other psychological variables are intervening, thus indirectly fostering recovery through the activation of the immune system to fight illness.

Another factor not yet clear in the study of humor and physiological systems is the role of laughter. As noted above, many of the benefits reported were in association with periods of laughter. Does laughter need to emerge during the humorous experience in order to mobilize the physiological systems of the body?

Yet another question for investigation relates to amounts of laughter or humor exposure needed to accomplish favorable results. It has been determined that frequent and continuous exercise–about 30 minutes, four to five times a week–is beneficial for the heart (McDowell, 1983). Is there a prescriptive formula for humor and laughter as well? How much of a "good thing" is needed? Are there prerequisites in order to benefit from it? As in the study above, do individuals need to have a high appreciation of humor to fully benefit from it?

Psychological Benefits of Humor

Williams (1986) points to four areas where humor is effective in producing psychic healing. The author states that humor provides: "(a) a relaxed atmosphere, (b) an escape outlet, (c) methods of communication, and (d) self-insight" (p 15). Robinson (1977) suggested five ways in which humor can be helpful in dealing with patients: (a) by releasing anger or hostility in socially acceptable ways, (b) by providing an opportunity for denial of frightening feelings, (c) by facilitating adjustment to new environments or circumstances, (d) by developing interpersonal relationships, and (e) by relieving anxiety and stress. She writes:

> Humor is a coping mechanism to relieve anxiety, stress, and tension; an outlet for hostility and anger, an escape from reality and a means of lightening the heaviness of related crises, tragedy, chronic illness, disabilities and death. (1982, p. 116)

Indicators of positive psychological well being suggested by Neugarten (1974) are: (a) pleasure taken in everyday life activities, (b) evaluation of one's life as meaningful and acceptable, (c) feeling of success from achieving life goals, (d) positive self-image, and (e) happy and optimistic moods and attitudes.

These happy attitudes may be a prevalent area in which humor can play an important role. Ryff (1989) conducted a study of 171 middle aged and older adults. Participants were questioned about general life evaluations, past life experiences, conceptions of well-being, and views of the aging process. The findings indicated that individuals considered sense of humor as an index of well being and successful aging.

Fry (1982) reported that humor is not only opposed to negative emotions, but also positively correlated with desired emotions like joy, excitement, hope and playfulness. Robinson (1983) considers humor as "a means of lightening tragedy, the heaviness of crises, chronic illness, disabilities and death" (p 116). Researchers in the area of humor have pointed to its value in assisting individuals to adapt to life stresses and anxieties (Mindess, 1971; Peter & Dana, 1982; Fry, 1982; Goodman, 1983). It has indeed been identified as a coping mechanism (Robinson, 1977; Lefcourt & Martin, 1986; Simon, 1988).

Humor has also been attributed the potential to facilitate communication and social interaction (Peter & Dana, 1982; Blumenfield & Alpern, 1986; Williams, 1986). Humor is described as "a form of indirect communication that covers messages that are usually emotionally tinged, and might be unacceptable if expressed or acknowledged directly" (Robinson, 1970).

In a study of 101 volunteer subjects of various ages and backgrounds, Fay (1983) utilized measures of stress (Schedule of Recent Events), anxiety (Personality Ability Testing Anxiety Scale), and appreciation of humor (Humor Appreciation Test) to examine the relationship between appreciation and utilization of humor and the ability to manage stress. Coping ability was determined by dividing scores on the stress inventory by scores on the anxiety test. Two groups were identified from the quotients obtained: effective copers, whose scores were two deviations above the mean and ineffective copers, whose scores were two deviations below the mean. The two groups were, then, compared in relation to their scores on a humor appreciation inventory. Results indicated that those subjects who were more capable to cope with life stress were also those more able to appreciate humor. Those less effective in dealing with stress showed less ability to utilize humor.

Martin and Lefcourt (1983) also found evidence regarding the moderating effect of humor over the impact of stressful life events on mood. Three studies were conducted. In the first study, a negative life events checklist to predict stress scores, a scale to assess mood and three different instruments to measure sense of humor were utilized with 56 university students as subjects. As hypothesized by the authors, the correlation between life stress and mood disturbance was significantly lower in those individuals scoring high on the sense of humor scales than those scoring low. In other words, as scores on the humor measures increased, a weaker relationship was found between negative events and depressed moods.

In the second study, 62 students were requested to complete the same measures as in study one. This time, a more behavioral measure of humor was utilized. After completion, subjects were asked to make up a three minute comedy routine describing objects placed on their tables. Recordings of their routines were made. A panel of judges rated the funniness of their routines by analyzing the number of witty remarks and overall wittiness judged on a five point scale. As with the other study, high scores in the behavioral measure of sense of humor contributed to a low relationship between stress and mood disturbance. Subjects who were able to produce a humorous routine, were also found to exhibit mirth in a variety of situations, as measured by one of the humor measures.

In the final study, subjects were asked to produce a funny narrative while watching a stressful film. The results obtained again confirmed the moderating effects of humor on the relationship between stress and mood disturbance. Subjects who were able to create a humorous monologue were also those who tended to use humor to cope with real life stresses as measured by the Humor Coping Scale.

A study by Porterfield (1987), however, revealed no evidence that humor moderates the impact of life stresses on depression or physical illness. The study, including 220 undergraduates, revealed that sense of humor directly reduced depression, independent of the effects of life events. These findings raise doubt concerning the previously hypothesized buffering effects of humor on the relationship between life events and mood, although it still offers support to the positive effect of humor on mood.

Other studies need to replicate the conditions of the above mentioned studies, controlling for other variables such as age, disposition for negative mood, types of negative stressors and levels of stress. Is it possible that a certain level of stress must exist before humor can buffer its effects on mood? Do some individuals show negative moods, regardless of the level of stress to which they are exposed? Are some stressors more likely to affect mood or to be affected by humor than others? Is it possible that a person with high appreciation of humor and utilization of humor as a coping device needs humor stimulation in order to take full advantage of its buffering effects? Or can it be assumed that appreciation and valuing of humor alone will lead to smaller risks regarding mood disturbance?

Mannel and McMahon (1982) documented the importance of humor to psychological well-being. Thirty-one university students were asked to keep a daily log in which they recorded the frequency and type of humorous experiences they had during a relatively normal day for them. For each humor encounter, subjects were supposed to indicate the source of the humorous experience, whether or not laughter had occurred and the level of amusement rated on a five-point scale.

Three copies of a mood adjective checklist were also included with the diary, with instructions for subjects to fill out one after waking up, one at noon, and one before going to bed at night. The relationship between changes in mood and humorous encounters were examined by correlating mood scores with number of humorous stimuli, overt laughs, and average amount of amusement reported. Results of the analysis of logs indicated that increases in positive moods and decreases in negative moods were significantly associated with higher incidence of humor and laughter.

One question raised by the author was: "Does humor indeed increase positive moods or does increase in positive mood from other sources account for enhanced perception of humor stimuli in the environment?" Research utilizing pretest measures of mood are necessary in order to determine if exposure to humor stimuli can indeed increase positive moods. Also measures such as those on appreciation of and coping with humor should be included to explain individual differences.

Nemeth (1979), studying the role of humor in reducing anxiety, assigned 75 patients awaiting medical treatment to one of three groups: (a) a group who was shown a silent humorous film, (b) a group who watched a silent non-humorous movie, and (c) a control group who watched no movies but remained in the waiting room for 30 minutes while the other two groups watched movies. Each group was administered the Institute for Personality Ability Testing Anxiety Scale prior to and following showing of the movies. The other instrument administered was the Preference Survey Questionnaire, designed by the researcher for rating the funniness of the movies by a panel of experts. The panel rated the film *Big Business* as the funniest of the four classic comedies viewed, thus recommending it for utilization in the study. Results of this experiment indicated that the group who watched the humorous movie had significantly lower levels of anxiety than the other two groups, who showed no significant reduction in anxiety. The study also showed that the subjects in the humor group reduced their anxiety levels to those experienced by the "general" population as indicated by comparison of means.

In discussing the implications of the study, Nemeth asks: "Would more exposure to non-threatening humor on a regular basis provide the individual with enough insights to help him overcome high anxieties and be able to better cope with his daily life?" (p. 43). This question merits further investigation. Can humor alleviate anxiety on a regular basis? Does it matter what the source of anxiety is, how acute or chronic it is? Can other humor modalities produce the same beneficial effects? Can anyone benefit from exposure to humor during anxiety-producing events? Can humor minimize the impact of high anxiety events such as transition into an institutional setting? Or does its effectiveness oscillate with the intensity of anxiety generated by the event as perceived by the subject?

A study by Lefcourt and Martin (1986) was designed to examine adaptation to physical disability in individuals ranging from age 18 to 78 years. Reactions to exposure to disability-related cartoons were recorded. Those disabled individuals who could laugh at cartoons were also found to be better functioning, demonstrating more vitality and higher self-concept.

If being able to laugh at one's own misfortune is a successful way to adapt, development of a sense of humor in individuals with disabilities should be encouraged. Can someone, though, be taught to use humor as a coping mechanism? Is the ability to use humor related to other variables already different in both groups–the well adapted and the poorly adapted–even before disability occurred? Can these other variables, rather than humor itself, explain the differences in adaptation? Could it be that vitality and self-concept were already higher in the well adapted persons, leading them to use humor more often, even prior to disability? Only longitudinal studies can answer this last question.

In the book *Adaptation to Life*, George Vaillant (1977) reported the results of a 30 year longitudinal study of 268 Caucasian male Harvard graduates from the classes of 1939 to 1944. At the time the subjects were selected for the study, all of them had achieved good academic standing and were judged to be healthy. In fact, college deans were asked to select subjects who were ''the most independent and who were less likely to come to the attention of medical services'' (p. 31). The focus of the study was on how these men adapted to life in areas such as work and how they stood in social, psychological and medical areas. After being accepted in the study, subjects were interviewed by psychiatrists, psychologists, sociologists, anthropologists and physicians. Several tests were administered, from electroencephalograms to the Scholastic Aptitude Test.

The subjects were reinterviewed during 1950-1952, their developmental histories being recorded and new tests run. Then, 30 years after the beginning of the study, Vaillant chose a sample of 100 subjects from the original group to be interviewed for the third time. From analyzing the lives of the subjects in the study, Vaillant identified humor as one of five mature coping mechanisms available to humans for coping with unfavorable circumstances. He stated:

> Humor is one of the truly elegant defenses of the human repertoire. Few would deny that the capacity of humor, like hope, is one of mankind's most potent antidotes to the woes of the Pandora's box. (p. 116)

As noted before, in the field of humor there is a great scarcity of longitudinal studies. Researchers rely on retrospective self-report on the utilization of humor during a lifetime, but have no way of confirming if indeed those who value and use humor during stressful times are more likely to avoid threats to psychological well-being. Can humor actually explain why some elderly individuals appear less affected by life stressors than others? How is humor molded throughout the lifespan? Can it be introduced in the later years or is it permanently shaped by the time one reaches old age?

Simon (1988) conducted a study with 24 adults, aged 61 to 89 years of age from a senior citizen community center in a large Texas city. Subjects were invited to participate; those who volunteered were administered questionnaires on current perceived health (Current Health Subscale), situational and coping humor (Situational Humor Response Questionnaire and Coping Humor Scale), life satisfaction (Life Satisfaction Index) and affect (Affect Balance Scale). The purpose of the study was to examine the relationship between the uses of humor and health outcomes, as measured by perceived health, life satisfaction and morale. The study revealed a positive relationship between situational humor (measured by an 18 item questionnaire and defined as frequency with which an individual displays mirth in a wide variety of life situations) and perceived health and morale. It also yielded a negative correlation between coping through humor (measured by a seven-item scale created to assess the degree to which an individual reports using humor to cope with stress) and health perception.

This study is particularly interesting because it utilizes elderly subjects as its sample. The fact that coping with humor was negatively correlated with perceived health was explained by the author as an indication that humor may be a coping strategy used only when there are health problems. Is it possible that the coping aspect of humor is activated only when the human body signals its low capacity to handle stress? Can humor, then, alert the immune system to protect the body from illness? Simon's study was limited in its sample size. Replications with larger and more diversified samples are needed to further investigate this intriguing result.

Miles (1988) conducted a study with 60 non-institutionalized adults 60 years old or older. The goal of the study was to determine if higher humor appreciation scores would be positively correlated with higher life satisfaction, functional health, self-esteem, and lower death anxiety. No significant results were found. Appreciation of humor was measured by a paper and pencil test in which subjects were asked to rate 50 jokes and cartoons on a five point scale ranging from "like the joke very much" to "do not like the joke at all." This instrument differed from the ones used in the studies discussed above in that it measured appreciation of some forms of humor stimulation at a given moment, not taking into consideration habitual appreciation or use of humor as a coping device. Other factors such as the present affect of the subjects may have influenced the ratings, thus interfering with the correlations with the dependent variables. More stable measures of sense of humor are needed if research is to uncover general trends regarding appreciation and utilization of humor and measures of psychological well-being. Also, consistency in the instrumentation is needed in order for results to be compared and generalized.

Peter and Dana (1982) report a three month experimental study in a convalescent home, in which a group met for 15 minutes daily, five times a week. Each day a different member of the group was responsible for the selection of humorous material. Each session also included joke telling by the leader. At the completion of the study, the researcher findings showed that there was: (a) more mirth, (b) more interaction, (c) less complaining, (d) sociability, (e) more alertness, and (f) more interest in personal appearance.

What is not clear from looking at the results of this study is whether the joke telling by the leader or the materials presented by the residents (or both) accounted for behavioral changes. The fact that residents were given the responsibility to bring humorous materials to the sessions incorporates a new variable into the research of the benefits of humor to psychological well-being. Is it reasonable to assume that added benefits can be expected if subjects are encouraged to seek humor stimuli they appreciate rather than being exposed to stimulation selected by others? Is it also possible that by making others laugh, extra feelings of control and efficacy contribute to raise morale, self confidence and socialization? Researchers should pay close attention to the manipulation of humorous stimuli when developing interventions. Variables that enhance or hinder the effectiveness of humor need to be identified and controlled.

A study conducted by the Ethel Percy Andrus Gerontology Center at the University of Southern California (Ewers et al., 1983) had similar results. A program called "Life Enrichment Through Humor in Long Term Care Facilities" was implemented in cooperation with the staff of a Los Angeles nursing hospital. The program incorporated a variety of approaches to introduce humor into the nursing home environment. A task force of volunteers composed by site personnel and students was used to run the program. Sixty residents were selected to participate in the project. Among the activities were singalongs of familiar songs, showings of old comedies and thematic parties. Although scientific evaluation was not possible due to difficulties in data gathering, observations kept of participants' behavior revealed some promising benefits.

Some of the behavioral changes observed included: (a) greater awareness of each other, (b) anticipation of the coming of program leaders, (c) expressed appreciation of the program, (d) enjoyment in discussing previous program days, (e) increased socialization, (f) expression of more outgoing attitudes, (g) initiation of programs by participants, (h) indication of enjoyment through smiles and laughter, (i) increased sense of humor in interactions with others, (j) greater openness to participation, and, (k) warm responses to volunteers. From the study, a handbook on how to infuse humor into long term care was developed.

For this study, a rather comprehensive intervention was developed. Several opportunities for humor exposure were created. An environmental approach rather than a single source of stimulation may be preferred. But it is necessary to know which sources are the most effective. Combinations of sources need to be tested in the future. As volunteers were used for the project, it is not safe to assume that humor alone brought about the positive changes reported. This point reinforces the notion that experimental designs need to employ control measures in order to increase internal validity. Or, if two variables are being analyzed conjunctively, statistical procedures need to be utilized to determine their separate and combined effects.

Napora (1984) investigated the relationship between activity and subjective well-being in older adults. To do so, the researcher conducted a program of humorous activity for a period of six weeks with 60 subjects, half participating in the humorous activity program and half serving as controls. Subjects involved in the experimental group showed elevated mood levels in association with humorous activity.

Napora's study did not use only humor activity as the dependent variable distinguishing both groups. Group participation itself may have affected the results, although humorous activity seemed to produce more elevated moods. Simple novelty may have played a role in the study. Again, the need for control of other intervening variables is an issue. Also, since most experimental interventions are done in group situations, more single-subject designs are needed to understand the impact of humor on subjects individually.

A recent study by Adams and McGuire (1986) explored the role of humor in reducing pain and increasing positive affect in residents of a long term care facility. Thirteen residents were assigned to either a humor group–who viewed humorous movies–or a serious group–who viewed non-humorous movies. After a six-week period, those subjects in the humor group showed higher levels of positive affect than those in the serious group, with no significant differences having been found in the affect measure in the pretest. Also, examination of changes in pain medication requests over the course of the study indicated a decrease in requests for all members of the experimental group while for only 50% of those in the serious group.

Adams and McGuire found significant results with a small sample, using one single facility. The next logical step seems to be to increase sample size and the extension of the study into different long term facilities in order to find out if the findings can be reproduced. Other questions such as variations in movie types and viewing schedules should also be taken into consideration. Is humor interacting with reminiscence in bringing about positive results? Does individual appreciation of humor affect the relationship between exposure to humorous stimuli and mood or perception of pain? Can other simple forms of stimulation work as well? For how long can the same source of stimulation be effective?

The studies presented above, although exploring different potential benefits of humor, point the way to necessary research into the relationship between humor and variables associated with quality of life.

Building on previous research, the study described in the next chapter was designed with the purpose of examining the effectiveness of humor in improving quality of life of residents of long term care facilities. Because of their relevance to old age, measures selected as indicators of life quality were pain reduction, adaptation and affect.

Humor has been approached in numerous ways in the past. To operationalize this multi-faceted construct, a simple intervention was devised, utilizing comic movies as the humorous stimuli. In order to increase confidence in the individual effect of humor as opposed to mere novelty or stimulation introduced by the presentation of movies, serious movies were also shown to a second group. A third group, used as a control, was not shown any movies.

If exposure to readily accessible forms of humor stimuli, such as comedies, produces beneficial effects on measures of physical and psychological well-being, the effort to build a more humorous environment is worthwhile for those serving nursing home residents. Humor may not be the solution to all problems faced by older adults, but it has the potential to stir up dormant emotions and introduce vital stimulation lacking in institutional settings. Further research is needed not only to confirm the hypothesis that humor can be therapeutic, but also to explore how and why humor might help fight boredom and improve the quality of life of older adults in long term care facilities.

The literature examined above provides support for the use of humor in long term care facitilies. There is strong evidence that humor can be an efficacious addition to the activity therapy program. The chapter which follows provides additional support for building a case for the serious role of humor in therapy.

Chapter III

The Clemson Humor Project

In the spring of 1989 a large scale study was conducted by the Department of Parks, Recreation and Tourism Management at Clemson University to determine whether exposure to humorous stimulation was an effective intervention in improving the quality of life of residents in long term care facilities. The vehicles used for introducing humor into the facilities cooperating in the project were movies. Indicators of quality of life used in the study were: happiness, adaptation, perceived health, and pain medication requests. The methods, results and conclusions of this project, known as the Clemson Humor Project, will be described in this chapter.

METHODS

Subjects

A major corporation located in South Carolina was contacted and agreed to participate in this study. The administrators and activity directors of the facilities operated by the corporation were contacted and the project was explained to them. A total of eight facilities responded positively to the invitation to join the study. Three facilities were located in South Carolina and eight in North Carolina. The facilities ranged in size from 62 beds to 192 beds. Each facility had an activity director and all contacts between the researchers and the facilities were made through the activity director. The activity director at each site was given the responsibility for the actual conduct of the study. This was done to determine whether the benefits expected would occur without the intervention of outside agents such as the researcher. It was felt that the humor intervention, to be truly effective, had to be successful within the staffing patterns of the facilities and without the addition of staff.

Each facility was requested to submit a list of the names of 30 residents who met the following requirements for inclusion in the study: the individual must have experienced chronic pain for at least six months, the individual must not have been scheduled for any medical or surgical procedures, the individual must have been alert and oriented, the individual must have agreed to participate in the study and complete all human subject procedures. From the lists submitted by the activity directors, subjects were randomly assigned to one of three groups: humorous, serious, and control. After placement into groups, all subjects were read a statement requesting their participation in the study and asked to sign a human subject informed consent form. A total of 234 individuals joined the project at its initiation. However, by the completion of the project 86 of these remained in the study. The reasons for the large drop-out rate will be discussed later.

The Humor Intervention

The type of humor stimulation selected for this project was comic movies. Thus, individuals assigned to the humorous group were shown humorous movies while those in the non-humorous group were shown movies with little humor content, such as dramas, mysteries, or westerns. The control group did not watch any movies unless they had been programmed for all residents as part of the normal activity program.

Based on previous research (Adams & McGuire, 1986) and a pilot project done at two long term care facilities, a list of movies identified as humorous by residents of these facilities was developed. Each activity director was mailed this list and asked to indicate which films were available in their local video store. The responses from the activity directors made it apparent that the researchers' desire for uniformity in movies shown by all facilities would not be possible since all the films were not available at each site. A final list reflecting the movies most frequently identified as available by the activity directors was developed and distributed to the eight facilities. The activity directors were instructed to utilize movies from the list in the program. They were also instructed to match the serious movies shown with the humorous movies in terms of length, period, and color. This was done to control for the effects of these extraneous variables.

Some activity directors found their residents had seen several of the movies on the list and did not want to see them again. Since the main concern regarding the movies was that they be entertaining, the activity directors were told to use their best judgment in selecting movies. As a result, the final selection of movies differed from the list originally provided. Allowing each facility to make the final choice of films resulted in each site showing a somewhat different list of films. Appendix A provides a list of all the movies used in this project.

Previous research indicated sessions of 40 minutes to one hour were appropriate for the humor/non-humor intervention. Therefore it was decided that both movie groups would be shown movies during sessions that did not exceed one hour, even if this meant having to watch an entire movie over two sessions. The activity directors were asked to select three days a week to show the humorous films and three days to show the serious films. The study was conducted over a 12 week period. In order to make sure any changes in participants were not the result of the timing of the films, activity directors were asked to switch times of films at the sixth week, thus giving a chance for those who had been watching films in the morning to do so in the afternoon and vice-versa.

Activity directors were gathered at a training session to familiarize them with the instruments to be used in the study. Each director was asked to rehearse administering the instruments prior to the beginning of the data gathering phase of the study. They also received written instructions concerning what to do each week of the study. They were told only that the study was developed to investigate strategies for implementing recreation programs in long term care facilities. During the conduct of the study, activity directors were called on a weekly basis and each director was visited by the researchers at least once during the study. They also received periodic mailings with forms and instructions throughout the study.

Prior to the showing of films, pretesting was conducted utilizing the Affect Balance Scale, the VIRO Scale, and a self-perceived health scale. In addition, a baseline measure of pain relief medication requests was obtained from nursing personnel at this time. The following section describes these instruments in greater detail.

After viewing each film, participants were asked to rate each movie on its funniness, for humorous movies, or entertainment value, for serious movies, on a three point scale ranging from "not funny/entertaining" to "very funny/entertaining." They were also asked to identify their frequency of laughter during each film from "not at all" to "often." Finally, the participants were asked to use a three point scale, ranging from "no better than before" to "much better than before," to indicate how the movie made them feel.

After the twelve weeks of the program, posttesting was conducted using the same measures as used on the pretest. In addition, pain medication request counts were collected from the participants' medical charts on a weekly basis during the study.

Data Gathering Instruments

A variety of instruments were used to gather the data which were analyzed to determine the effectiveness of humor in this project. The following is a description of these.

Pain. A record sheet was developed with the dates of each of the 12 weeks of the study, as well as the week immediately preceding and following this 12 week period. Nurses were instructed to use each participant's medical chart to provide a count of the number of analgesic requests for each of the 14 weeks. The week ran from 12:01 Sunday to midnight Saturday. The requests were used as an indicator of the experience of pain by each participant. It was assumed that decreases in pain would be accompanied by decreases in requests for pain relief medication.

Self-Reported Health. After examination of several health perception measures, the Health Perception Questionnaire (Ware, 1976) was selected and adapted for use in this study. The original instrument had 36 items. Five of these were used in the study. These five were selected because of their representativeness of the areas covered in the original questionnaire. A four point scale, ranging from "strongly disagree" to "strongly agree," was used with each question. The five items used in this study were:

1. My physical health has been excellent the past two weeks;
2. I have experienced a great deal of pain in the past two weeks;
3. I will probably be sick a lot in the future;
4. I have been feeling quite depressed in the past two weeks;
5. I have not been worried about my health lately.

Each item was considered separately for analysis purposes and no attempt was made to extract one general health score from these items since no reliability testing was done. The original 36 items questionnaire was reduced since it was believed the lengthier instrument, in conjunction with the other instrument used in this study, would have been overly taxing on the respondents. Participants were given the health questionnaire at the time of the pretest and posttest interview and asked to complete it before the end of the week during which testing took place. Scoring was done by assigning a value of 1 to a "strongly disagree" response, a 2 to "mildly disagree," a 3 to "mildly agree," and a 4 to "strongly agree." Items 1 and 5 are positive statements and therefore a high score was indicative of a positive perception of health. Items 2, 3 and 4 are negatively worded with high scores indicating a negative health perception.

Happiness. The measure selected to measure happiness in this study was the Affect Balance Scale (ABS) developed by Bradburn (1969). According to the developer, the ABS measures happiness which "is the degree to which a person's positive feelings about life outweigh his negative feelings" (George & Bearon, 1980).

The ABS is composed of 120 items, five indicating a positive affect and five indicating negative affect. Respondents are expected to answer "yes" or "no" to a series of questions about feelings they have experienced in the past few weeks. Items are phrased in general terms since the concern in the instrument is not with the content of the experience but rather with its pleasurable or unpleasureable character (Sauer & Warland, 1982). The opening statement of the ABS states: "During the past two weeks did you ever feel . . ." and this is followed by five positive statements such as "that things were going your way" and five negative statements such as "bored."

The scale was administered during a structured interview in this project. The activity director read the items to each respondent and recorded responses.

Scoring was done by assigning a value of one to each "yes" response and 0 to each "no" response. The scores on the five positive items were summed to yield a positive affect score. This score could therefore range from one to five, with a five being the highest possible positive affect score. The scores for the five negative items were also summed. In this case, a total score of five indicated the highest possible negative affect score. The negative affect score was then subtracted from the positive affect score, and a constant of five was then added to this score, to provide an overall score. The constant was used to ensure no scores would be negative. The total ABS score, therefore, ranged from 0 (low total affect) to 10 (high affect).

The reliability of the ABS was reported by Bradburn (1969) to be .76. Bradburn (1969) indicated that the proportion of scores changing over time is much higher than what would be expected based on the reliability estimates. This indicates how susceptible affect is to change.

According to Bradburn (1969) the two dimensions of affect are distinct. Positive affect is correlated with measures of social participation, degree of sociability and companionship with spouse, and exposure to situations introducing variability to life. Contrarily, negative affect was found to correlate primarily with variables indicating maladjustment, such as interpersonal tensions, anxiety, worry, and difficulties adjusting to work and marriage. Moriwaki (1974) corroborated Bradburn's findings in a study of elderly individuals. She found the positive scale to be correlated with morale and happiness and the negative scale to be correlated with poor health. Further research by Mangen (1977) confirmed the presence of two distinct orthogonal dimensions in this scale.

Adaptation. The instrument used to measure adaptation was the VIRO Scale. VIRO stands for vigor, intactness, relationships, and orientation. Although the scale does not focus directly on assessing coping behavior, many of the behaviors it assesses are related to this concept (Kahana, Fairchild, & Kahana, 1982).

Vigor is defined as "the energy level manifested by the subject during the course of the interview." Intactness represents "cognitive aspects of the subject's interview behavior in terms of maintaining a conversation within the social context." Relationship refers to " the measure and style of interacting with the interviewer." Orientation is "a measure of cognitive functioning as assessed by direct questioning concerning time, place, and interview content" (Kastenbaum & Sherwood, 1972, p. 181).

The VIRO Scale consists of 21 items scored on a four point scale. Each item contributes to only one of the four dimensions of the scale. The higher the score, the more desirable it is considered to be. The maximum scores for vigor, intactness, relationship, and orientation are 6, 15, 15, and 14 respectively.

Administration of the scale is done through interviewing subjects and rating their responses according to the bipolar dimensions provided. Bipolar dimensions include items such as "vigorous vs. feeble" for vigor, "keen attention vs. poor attention" for intactness, and "eager participation vs. reluctant participation" for relationship. Orientation is based on items such as "knows community" and "knows age."

In order to provide a uniform structure to all interviews used to complete the VIRO Scale, the activity directors were asked to use the questions on the ABS as the main topic of conversation. They were also requested to administer the orientation questions after the affect related questions.

The VIRO Scale is useful in establishing baseline behavior before introduction of an intervention and in measuring treatment outcomes following intervention (Kastenbaum & Sherwood, 1972). Kahana et al. (1982) indicated it was suitable for older populations and was developed for use in a wide range of situations. Therefore, it was deemed to be an appropriate tool for use in the Clemson Humor Project.

Data Analysis

Several individuals who originally agreed to participate in the study were unable to attend all the sessions of the program. It was decided to limit the analysis to individuals who had watched at least

12 movies during the course of the study. This was done to assure data be gathered only from individuals whose participation was at a level sufficient to bring about the expected changes.

Paired t-tests were used to determine whether respondents within groups experienced significant changes from pretest to posttest on affect, perceived health, and adaptation. Pain medication requests were traced along the 14 weeks of data gathering through comparison of repeated ANOVAs for each week and t-tests of consecutive weeks. Analysis of Covariance, with pretest scores as the covariate in the analysis, was used in examining between group changes in affect, perceived health and adaptation. The Mann-Whitney U Test was used to determine whether the groups differed in how they felt after watching each movie, as well as in frequency of laughter. Chi square analysis was used to determine whether there was a relationship between the amount of laughter reported by a respondent and the extent to which the respondent reported feeling better. Descriptive statistics were used to determine which movies were rated as the funniest by participants in the humor group.

Due to the exploratory nature of the study, it was decided to use .10 as the acceptable level of significance. Although this is higher than in many studies, the danger of rejecting relationships which may actually exist was viewed as more deleterious than accepting relationships which were actually chance occurrences. Any findings significant at the more rigorous .05 level are noted in the text.

RESULTS

The Clemson Humor Project was designed to determine whether humor was efficacious in achieving therapeutic benefits in residents of long term care facilities. The results of this project are reported in the following section.

Subjects

The initial sample included 234 participants. However, problems resulting from incomplete or not returned forms and drop-outs from the study, resulted in a decision to limit the study to those respondents viewing and completing information for at least 12 movies. (This level of involvement was selected because it was the average attendance level of participants.)

The final sample for this study included 86 subjects, 27 in the humor group, 18 in the non-humor group and 41 in the control group. All the participants did not provide all the requested information. As a result, all 86 were not included in all analyses. These participants came from four of the original eight facilities agreeing to be in the study. The four facilities withdrawing from the study did so for a variety of reasons. The activity director in one facility left and the project ended at that time. A second facility allowed participants to watch any movie and did not retain the concept of limiting the humor and non-humor groups to only the designated movie type. The other two facilities did not show movies regularly and therefore no resident watched 12 or more films.

Of the 86 subjects considered for analysis, the mean age was 80.42. The average length of stay in the facility was 39.06 months. Approximately 72% were females, and the average number of movies watched was 21.9.

The humor group had a mean age of 83.5 years and mean length of stay of 30 months. It was 92.3% female and the average number of movies watched was 20.8. The non-humor group had a mean age of 79.6 and an average length of stay of 46.5 months. Approximately 72% of this group were female and they watched an average of 23.6 movies. The control group had an average age of 78.7, with a mean length of stay of 41.9 months. This group was more balanced than the other two in terms of gender, with 59% of the group members being females. Members of this group viewed no movies.

Analyses were done to determine whether the differences among the groups on the background variables were significant. The only variable which varied significantly (chi square = 8.5, p = .01) across the three groups was gender. Therefore, gender was included as a variable in data analysis as appropriate.

The Impact of Humor on Affect

Comparison of the pretest and posttest scores on the Affect Balance Scale of the humor group was done to determine whether there was a change in affect over the course of the study. Similar comparisons were made for the serious and the control groups. (See Table 1.) None of the groups experienced a significant ($p < .10$) change in positive affect from the pretest to the posttest. However, the humor group was the only one of the three which exhibited an increase in positive affect during the study.

All three groups displayed a significant ($p < .05$) decrease in negative affect during the twelve weeks of the study. It was surprising that even the control group, who experienced no change in their daily routine would display a decrease in the amount of negative affect they experienced.

The total affect score, obtained by subtracting negative affect from positive affect and adding a constant of 5, was also examined for all three groups. Two groups experienced a significant ($p < .10$) change from pretest to posttest in total affect. The humor group experienced a significant ($p < .05$) increase in affect, from a score of 5.77 at the pretest to 7.14 at the time of the posttest. The control group also increased significantly ($p < .10$) in total affect, from 5.20 to 5.94.

Although the results of these t-tests are of interest, they do not indicate which, if any, between group differences were significant after the treatment phase of the study. According to Campbell and Stanley (1963) the use of analysis of covariance with pretest scores as covariates is a desirable approach to such an analysis. Therefore, between group comparisons on affect scores was done using analysis of covariance. Table 2 presents the results of this analysis.

The examination of between group differences in positive affect indicated a significant ($p < .05$) difference existed between the groups on posttest positive affect after removing differences explained by pretest differences between the group. Further analysis, using Duncan's test, resulted in the conclusion that the difference was between the posttest scores of the humor and control group. The humor group had significantly higher posttest scores than the control group. Although the humor group's posttest scores were higher than those of the serious group, this difference was not significant ($p > .10$).

The analysis of posttest differences on negative affect indicated there were no between group posttest differences. The groups were

Table 1

Results of Within Group T-Tests Pretest to Posttest Scores for

Affect

Variable	Group					
	Humor		Serious		Control	
	Pretest Mean	Posttest Mean	Pretest Mean	Posttest Mean	Pretest Mean	Posttest Mean
Total Affect	5.77	7.13**	5.76	6.23	5.20	5.94*
Positive Affect	3.13	3.50	3.17	3.00	2.85	2.54
Negative Affect	2.36	1.36**	2.41	1.76**	2.65	1.60**
Vigor	4.16	4.75*	4.58	4.94	3.81	4.27
Relation- ship	11.91	12.08	13.29	13.88	12.84	12.36
Intact- ness	11.45	12.33*	12.64	13.35	12.05	12.41
Orienta- tion	8.33	9.16	10.76	11.94**	10.26	10.44
H 1 (a)	3.19	3.19	3.07	3.15	2.84	2.71
H 2	1.80	2.09	2.26	2.60	2.35	2.35
H 3	1.90	1.57	1.80	1.73	2.20	1.94
H 4	2.00	2.33	2.40	1.45	2.11	1.71*
H 5	2.95	2.85	2.20	2.13	2.20	2.45

* $p < .10$

** $p < .05$

(a) H 1 My physical health has been excellent the past two weeks.

H 2 I have experienced a treat deal of pain in the past two weeks.

H 3 I will probably be sick a lot in the future.

H 4 I have been feeling quite depressed in the past two weeks.

H 5 I have not been worried about my health lately

Table 2

Between Group Differences of Affect and VIGOR Posttests Using

Pretest Scores as a Covariate

Variable	Adjusted Means			Group Differences
	Humor	Serious	Control	
Positive Affect	3.47	2.96	2.57	Humor & Control**
Negative Affect	1.42	1.89	1.53	None
Total Affect	7.01	6.11	6.07	Humor & Control*
Vigor	4.73	4.76	4.38	None
Relationship	12.59	13.49	12.22	Serious & Control*
Intactness	12.58	13.05	12.38	None
Orientation	10.20	10.07	10.05	None
H 1 (a)	3.13	3.14	2.75	None
H 2	2.18	2.57	2.30	None
H 3	1.59	1.77	1.90	None
H 4	2.39	2.42	1.73	Humor & Control*/ Serious & Control*
H 5	2.98	2.07	2.39	Humor & Serious*/ Humor & Control*

* $p < .10$

** $p < .05$

(a) H 1 My physical health has been excellent the past two
         weeks.

     H 2 I have experienced a treat deal of pain in the past two
         weeks.

     H 3 I will probably be sick a lot in the future.

     H 4 I have been feeling quite depressed in the past two
         weeks.

     H 5 I have not been worried about my health lately

equivalent on their posttest scores when controlling for pretest scores.

The final analysis related to affect examined the between group differences on total affect posttest scores. No significant differences were found. However, the main effect for group approached significance ($p = .15$). Therefore, Duncans' test was used to examine each pair of groups to determine if differences existed. The control and humor group differed ($p < .10$) on their posttest scores, with the humor group having significantly higher total affect.

The Impact of Humor on Adaptation

Scores on the 4 dimensions of the VIRO scale were examined within each group. T-tests were used to determine whether significant differences existed in the pretest and posttest scores of each group. As can be seen in Table 1 the humor group experienced significant changes ($p < .10$) in vigor and intactness. In both cases, the mean score on these dimensions improved from the pretest to the posttest. The serious group exhibited significant improvement on orientation between the pretest and posttest.

An analysis of covariance was done to examine whether significant posttest differences existed between the groups while controlling for pretest differences. The results indicated that only one dimension of the VIRO Scale, relationship, approached significance ($p = .108$). The difference in posttest scores was between the serious and the control group, with the serious group exhibiting a significantly ($p < .10$) higher relationship score. These results are presented in Table 2.

The Impact of Humor on Self-Perceived Health

The change from pretest to posttest for the three groups on each of the five health questions was also examined. As can be seen in Table 1 the only significant change was in the control group's responses to the question related to feeling depressed. They indicated decreased levels of depression over the course of the study.

Analysis of covariance for the health related question yielded some between group differences. Responses to question 1 ("My physical health has been excellent lately''), question 2 (''I have experienced a great deal of pain lately'') and question 3 (''I'll probably be sick a lot in the future'') were not related to group membership. Question 4 (''I have been feeling quite depressed in the past two weeks'') did exhibit group differences. The control group's posttest scores were significantly lower ($p < .10$) than those of the humor or serious group. In this case a low score indicated lower levels of self-perceived depression. Responses to question 5 (''I have not been worried about my health lately'') also yielded significant ($p < .10$) between group differences. The humor group had a significantly higher score on this item than either of the other two groups. This indicated that the humor group was less worried about their health than either of the other two groups. (See Table 2.)

The Mediating Effect of Gender

Since the three groups were significantly different in their gender composition, the above analyses of covariance were repeated using the additional variable of gender as an independent variable. The results were slightly different from those found above. There was only one change in the relationships found between the dependent variables and group membership. The significant between group difference in positive affect was not found when gender was added to the analysis. However, the between group difference approached significance ($p = .129$).

The Impact of Humor on Pain

None of the analyses related to requests for medication indicated either significant changes within any group or significant differences between groups existed. There were no significant changes when examining requests from one week to the next. In addition, no changes were found when examining the medication requests at week 1 with those at week 14. Table 3 reports the weekly average number of medications taken by members of each group.

Table 3

Comparison of Average Weekly Medications For Humor, Serious and

Control Groups

	Average Number of Medication Requests		
Week	Humor Group	Serious Group	Control Group
1 (Baseline)	.7826	3.1111	1.2831
2	.5217	2.2778	1.2857
3	.7083	1.2222	1.3889
4	.7500	.6111	2.7500
5	.7917	.5000	.8286
6	.8333	.6111	.7714
7	1.0417	1.0000	.9143
8	.9167	.5000	.7714
9	.7500	.7778	.9143
10	.2174	.7222	3.2140
11	.1304	.6667	.1071
12	.3333	.7778	.7914
13	.2500	.8571	1.5128
14 (Posttest)	.5500	.9286	2.2308

The Impact of Humor on Feeling Better

At the conclusion of each film respondents were asked to indicate if they felt "no better than before," "better than before," or "much better than before." Data from this question were used to compare differences between the humor and serious group of perceptions immediately following the viewing of a movie. The Mann Whitney U Test was used to compare the groups on whether viewing each movie resulted in feeling better. Since different schedules were used at each facility, it was not possible to compare specific films. Rather the comparison was between type of film, humorous or serious. A total of 25 films were compared. Although some participants viewed more than 25 movies, group sizes were below 10 after this point. Therefore, only the first 25 films viewed were analyzed. Of these, there was a significant difference in feeling better for 8 of the 25 comparisons. In every case, the humor group reported feeling better than the serious group.

The Relationship Between Humorous Movies and Laughter

The intent of showing movies identified as humorous was, obviously, to introduce humor into the lives of viewers. Although a pilot study indicated the movies selected were in fact funny, it was felt further examination of this expectation was needed. Therefore, respondents viewing movies were asked to indicate how often they laughed during the film. It was expected that individuals watching humorous movies would laugh more often than individuals watching serious films. Participants were asked "How often did you laugh" at the completion of each film. Responses were "not at all" (scored as a 1), "sometimes" (scored as a 2), and "often" (scored as a 3). The mean laughter score for all humorous group films was 2.28 and for the serious group was 1.62. Therefore, the humor group experienced significantly ($p < .05$) more laughter than the serious group. This finding was supported when the group differences in laughter were compared for each film. The humor group exhibited significantly more laughter in 19 of the 25 comparisons.

The Relationship of Laughter to Feeling Better

The final analysis using the instrument completed immediately following each session of the program examined the relationship between laughter and feeling better. Answers to the question about frequency of laughter were crosstabulated with responses to the question about how respondents felt after watching the film. The responses to the "feeling better" question were collapsed into two categories: (1) no better than before; (2) better or much better than before. Chi square analysis was done to determine whether the extent of laughter was related to feeling better. In every instance, feeling better was closely associated with laughter. Analysis was completed for 20 film viewings. Beyond this point, the cell frequencies were too small for meaningful comparisons. Table 4 presents the results of this analysis.

Which Movies Are the Funniest

Responses to the request to rate the movies used in the humorous group are reported in Table 5. All humorous movies shown are listed in this table. The ratings of each of these films, on funniness and laughter, are also provided.

Among the films seen by many participants and rated as somewhat or very funny by a large percentage of viewers were: "I Love Lucy" (a variety of episodes were shown); "Amos & Andy" (a variety of episodes); "The Honeymooners" (a variety of episodes); and "The 3 Stooges" (various episodes).

CONCLUSIONS AND IMPLICATIONS

The purpose of the Clemson Humor project was to add to the body of literature related to the therapeutic efficacy of humor. The findings of the study were mixed. Clearly, humor can be beneficial to residents of long term care facilities. However, it is not a panacea which will be all things to all people. It is, rather, another tool at the disposal of the activity professional attempting to meet client needs.

Conclusions

1. Affect appears to be an area where humor may be an effective agent for change. Humor can provide an instrument for happiness and satisfaction with life. The findings indicate that the infusion of humor into the routine of long term care facilities has the ability to bring about dormant positive feelings. Watching serious movies did not appear to have the same result. Since the emotional component of life is a major factor in overall quality of life, this is an extremely meaningful finding. In fact, it alone is sufficient justification for the development of humor programs.

Table 4

Relationship between Amount of Laughter and Feeling Better

	Amount of Laughter					
	No Laughter		Some Laughter		Frequent Laughter	
	How Did the Film Make You Feel					
	No Better	Better	No Better	Better	No Better	Better
Film	%	%	%	%	%	%
1	86.8	13.2	15.1	84.9	15.0	85.0**
2	64.9	13.2	15.1	84.9	5.0	95.0**
3	89.7	10.3	38.3	61.7	7.7	92.3**
4	69.2	30.8	28.0	72.0	11.1	88.9**
5	96.0	4.0	31.9	68.1	0.0	100.0**
6	83.9	16.1	36.4	63.6	0.0	100.0**
7	67.9	32.1	29.4	70.6	0.0	100.0**
8	90.3	9.7	36.0	64.0	10.0	90.0**
9	91.3	8.7	25.0	75.0	12.5	87.5**
10	91.7	8.3	38.9	61.1	6.7	93.3**
11	76.2	23.8	19.0	81.0	0.0	100.0**
12	71.4	28.6	14.3	85.7	0.0	100.0**
13	81.2	18.2	0.0	100.0	7.7	92.3**
14	80.0	20.0	9.5	90.5	0.0	100.0**
15	70.0	30.0	16.7	83.3	0.0	100.0**
16	55.6	44.4	15.8	84.2	0.0	100.0**
17	50.0	50.0	13.3	86.7	0.0	100.0**
18	60.0	40.0	15.4	84.6	0.0	100.0**
19	62.5	37.5	7.1	92.9	14.3	85.7**
20	55.6	44.4	7.1	92.9	0.0	100.0**

** $p < .05$

Table 5

Participant Ratings of Humorous Movies

	Film Rating					
	How Funny Was This Film			How Much Did You Laugh		
Movie	Not Funny n	Somewhat Funny n	Very Funny n	Not At All n	Some n	Alot n
W.C Fields	0	1	4	0	1	4
Comedy Bag	0	3	1	0	12	3
Lucy	5	17	37	7	18	38
T.V. Commercial	0	2	4	0	2	4
Amos & Andy	9	73	19	13	60	29
Honeymooners	4	33	19	8	29	22
Laurel & Hardy	26	44	19	33	44	15
Flying Dudes	0	2	3	0	2	3
Going Out West	1	4	4	1	4	4
Volume 1	0	6	1	0	4	3
Room Service	0	6	4	1	7	2
Animal Crackers	3	3	2	3	5	0
3 Stooges	7	23	14	7	27	10
18 Again	4	7	3	3	11	4
Bowery Boys	1	3	5	1	8	2
Cocoon II	1	4	8	2	4	7
We're No Angels	0	6	8	2	9	3
Young at Heart	0	0	3	0	0	3
Touch of Mink	3	2	2	4	1	2
No Deposit, No Return	0	6	0	2	4	0
Kid With the Broken Halo	3	2	13	4	6	8
Mac & Me	2	20	2	0	21	3
Connecticut Yankee	0	14	4	3	12	3
It's a Wonderful Life	0	4	8	0	4	8

Table 5 (cont.)

Participant Ratings of Humorous Movies

	Film Rating					
	How Funny Was This Film			How Much Did You Laugh		
Movie	Not Funny n	Somewhat Funny n	Very Funny n	Not At All n	Some n	Alot n
Your Show of Shows	10	8	2	10	7	3
At War With the Army	5	4	0	8	13	0
The Clown	3	4	2	3	4	2
Mr. Mom	1	12	7	2	11	7
Harry & Hendersons	0	3	1	0	2	2
Hold That Ghost	3	3	0	4	2	0
Yours, Mine & Ours	6	19	4	15	15	2
The Kid	3	8	0	5	4	2
Candid Camera	7	0	0	7	0	0
Going Bananas	0	1	3	0	2	2
Incredible Mr. Linipet	0	3	0	0	2	1
Uncle Buck	1	4	0	3	6	1
Popeye	0	3	1	0	2	2
Honey I Shrunk the Kds	5	8	0	8	9	0
Disorderlies	0	10	1	0	7	4
Pee Wees Adventure	0	3	1	1	2	2
Funny Farm	0	4	2	0	3	3
Bohemian Girl	1	7	0	1	5	2
Return to Mayberry	0	9	0	0	6	3
Shakiest Gun in the West	0	3	3	0	2	4
Smokey & the Bandit	0	3	3	0	3	3

Film Rating

	How Funny Was This Film			How Much Did You Laugh		
Movie	Not Funny n	Somewhat Funny n	Very Funny n	Not At All n	Some n	Alot n
Abbott & Costello	2	8	2	2	6	4
Best of	1	5	2	0	6	1
Live	0	2	4	0	0	6
Jack & Beanstalk	0	2	2	0	2	2
African Screams	0	10	5	0	8	7
Meet the killer	0	2	2	0	1	4
Red Skelton	1	8	2	1	6	3
Stolen Jewels	0	3	3	1	4	1
Bob Hope	1	5	2	0	6	2
Road to Bali	5	10	11	8	16	10
My Fav. Brunette	1	1	1	5	1	1
Little Rascals	0	2	10	0	2	10
Turner and Hooch	2	6	0	2	6	0
Roger Rabbit	0	3	0	1	1	1

a - Not all participants rated all films in all categories

2. The findings of this study did not provide strong support for the expected benefits in the area of adaptation and adjustment. Data from the VIRO Scale were mixed. Comparisons within the humor group from pretest to posttest indicated they experienced improvement in vigor and intactness. However, the between group comparisons at the conclusion of the study did not support a conclusion that humor was an effective intervention in these areas.

3. In terms of self-perceived health, the results were also mixed. Although the individuals in the humor group appeared significantly less worried about their health at the conclusion of the study than members of the control group, they also exhibited more self-report-

ed depression. It may be that the humorous films were awakening memories about life prior to admission to the facility and as a result participants were unhappy with their environment. Tennant (1986) provided an alternate explanation for this finding. She indicated humor is a coping mechanism used by patients. She provided an example of humor being useful in reducing anxiety about the seriousness of one's illness. In the present study, humor may have reduced anxiety related to health.

4. The expected relationship between humor and pain reduction was not found. Several explanations for this are possible. The first is that humor may not be an effective analgesic. However, previous research seems to contradict this conclusion. An alternate explanation lies in the nature of respondents. In spite of the request that only participants experiencing pain be included in the project, many participants were requesting few pain relief medications. As a result, a floor effect may have been operating in the study. Simply put, there may have been little room for improvement.

5. Viewing humorous films resulted in "feeling better" at least in the short term. In addition, it appeared that the more one laughs the better one feels. Clearly, this supports the use of humor if for no other reason than it facilitates a feeling of well-being. Introducing a program to increase laughter and incorporating funny moments into the day may be an effective tool for dealing with anxiety.

Practical Implications

In this study, exposure to humor via movies appeared to have benefits for residents of long term care facilities. Previous research strengthens our belief that the findings are valid and reflect real benefits. A variety of activities are available for introducing humor into long-term care facilities. These are detailed in Chapter IV of this manuscript and will not be explicated here. The implications below relate directly to this study.

The use of film to introduce humor into long term care facilities is an inexpensive and readily available approach. However, it probably should be used with other approaches to maximize its effectiveness. It is recommended that movies be used as part of a comprehensive program of humor stimulation. The relatively limited positive results found in this study may have been greatly expanded with a more intensive program.

Care must be used in selecting the movies to be shown. Individuals may have very strong feelings relating to the content, language, plot and characterizations in films. For example, one participant in this study was offended by films featuring Amos and Andy. This could have been avoided if a prior assessment of interests and preferences had been done.

Humor may provide a motivating force which keeps individuals involved and active. For example, several activity directors indicated the dropout rate in this study was higher for the serious group than for the humor group. Although this is anecdotal information, it does provide an intriguing possibility of a benefit of humor which has not been the focus of much study. Using humor in programs may be an effective method of retaining participants' interest.

The rating of movies as funny provides some insight into what may be the most effective types of films to use in a humor movie program. Many individuals preferred old situation comedies over feature length movies. This may be as a result of the ease of showing old television shows in a one hour block of time. Feature length movies must either be viewed in a 90 minute to 2 hour block or shown over two days. Both of these approaches may result in dissatisfaction. It may also be that the old television shows, which were probably viewed many times during adulthood, precipitated reminiscing to a greater extent than feature films which may have been viewed never or only once during an earlier period in life.

Although the results of this study did not necessarily confirm that laughter is the best medicine, they did support its efficacy as a therapeutic modality from which at least some individuals will benefit. That serves as justification for both its inclusion in programs and further research. While it is not a panacea which will transform long term care facilities into comedy clubs where a good time is had by all, it may provide a link with the past, a grounding in the present, and a hope for the future. For example, participating in an "I Love Lucy" film festival may provide a trigger for reminiscing about the past. In addition it may provide a shared experience which is the basis for social interaction with other viewers in the facility and at the same time give participants something to look forward to as the festival extends over several days.

Limitations of the Study

The authors of this collection would be remiss if they did not acknowledge the limitations in this study. Incorporating a variety of facilities spread across two states into the study resulted in several potential problems. Using activity directors to gather data and lead programs may have resulted in biases based on their lack of formal research training. Using one trained researcher to do all the data gathering and programming would have resulted in stronger internal reliability. However, this would have been at the expense of external reliability. It was decided to use the activity director in each facility and provide as much training and monitoring as possible. Nevertheless, some activity directors did not follow all the suggested procedures. As a result caution is needed in interpreting the findings.

Since the same movies were not available to all facilities, there was variation in the films shown. It would have been preferable to use the same movies at each facility in order to reduce variability in movies shown. However, this was not practical. Nevertheless, forms completed by participants at the conclusion of each film indicated the movies were introducing humor as anticipated. Some of the movies shown to the humor and serious groups may not have been appropriate for the intended group.

Although attempts were made to keep activity directors and participants blind to the purpose of the study, the large amount of interest generated by the project, and resulting stories in newspapers and on television made this impossible. Radio, television and newspapers conducted interviews at several sites and it is likely these were observed by the individuals participating in the study. Knowledge of the intent of the study may have influenced the results, although that is not known.

The large drop out rate may have also influenced the results of this study. However, individuals were assured at the beginning of the study they could stop participating at any time. Therefore, this was an unavoidable reality which can easily occur in a study of the duration of this one.

A limitation related to the drop-out rate in this study was the difference in group compositions. The humor, control, and serious groups became more different in composition in terms of gender, race, age, and length of stay as participants left the study.

Nevertheless, the results of this study should provide sufficient evidence to support cautious implementation of humor programs. Further efforts to evaluate the efficacy of humor in therapy are also needed.

Chapter IV

Humor Techniques, Activities and Resources

This chapter will provide information on a variety of techniques and approaches to facilitating humor in long term care facilities. It will include descriptions of programs, information about blocks to humor, a humor assessment, and resources useful in developing a humor program.

There are people who laugh spontaneously, but most of them are in treatment. The rest of us rely on stimuli: our friend's review of her first day on the job, the boss's jokes, a momentary sighting of a reflection in the mirror, or even the self-directed suggestion that a laugh might be helpful in this situation. More and more helping professionals are enjoying the challenge of providing the stimuli, the sights, sounds, experiences, and recollections, that elicit laughter or draw a few grins.

The activities found herein are intended to effect outcomes in two areas. An activity is classified in the category of humor generation (intended to produce "ha ha's") or in the category of humor appreciation (intended to produce "aha's"). Not all activities in humor programs are meant to be funny. Some experiences are structured to help individuals explore their own senses of humor, to think about the kinds of things that are most funny to them. Other activities help clients identify personal and environmental constraints to laughter and ways in which these obstacles can be removed or circumvented. Activities can be arranged to heighten clients' awareness of the humor in daily events and provide ideas and a lab for practicing ways to exercise the sense of humor. Activities can even be used to gently convey to clients that, like virtually everything else in life, getting one's recommended daily allowance of laughter is the individual's responsibility.

EXEMPLARY PROGRAMS

Goodman's HUMOR Project

Joel Goodman (1983) founded the HUMOR Project as a mechanism to "(1) explore the nature and nurture of humor by helping people learn, practice and apply skills for tapping their own sense of humor; (2) to develop and disseminate practical uses of humor that managers, teachers, parents, helping professionals, business people, and young people could integrate into their own work and life-style" (p. 2). The HUMOR Project supports the development of humor through a variety of workshops, speeches, and training sessions. In addition, the quarterly journal *Laughing Matters* is published by them. The HUMOR Project is an excellent resource for developing humor programs. Their address is included in the resource list at the conclusion of this chapter.

Goodman (1983) identified what he views as the four key ingredients in humor. They are: (1) The Eye of the Behohoholder; (2) Discover the ELF in YoursELF; (3) Get With It; (4) Follow the rule of the 5 Ps.

The eye of the behohoholder. Goodman recognizes the presence of humor all around us. It may not always be obvious but it is there if you look. Go through a day looking for humor and make a list of what you see and hear. Goodman suggests wearing your "Candid Camera glasses" for five minutes each day and recording your observations. Goodman shares quotes from a teacher who kept a record of classroom flubs. These included statements such as: "A census taker is a man who goes from house to house increasing the population" and "Water is composed of two gins. Oxygin and Hydrogin. Oxygin is pure gin. Hydrogin is gin and water." Similar examples can be found in any setting. For example, a magazine called *The Lutheran* includes a regular section called "Lite Side." It reports amusing quotes from church bulletins and newsletters. A recent issue included:

Please bring an offering and a snake to share. This is a fun way to be actively involved in congregational ministry.

Nursery Remodeling–Thanks to the efforts of Circle #2, the nursery has been cleaned up and painted. What a wonderful wetness.

There will not be a Week of Prayer for Unity Service next Sunday, due to scheduling conflicts for five of the six congregations involved.

You as a spiritual leader in Sacramento are encouraged to attend, be robbed and participate in the procession.

Apparently church bulletins are a rich source of humor. Goodman cites several items similar to those above and similar items often appear in the *Reader's Digest*. Similar lists of flubs could be developed in a long term care facility and become the focal point of a bulletin board or newsletter. Residents as well as staff could become "flub detectives" seeking out humor in everyday occurrences.

The Elf in yoursElf. Goodman's second suggestion for developing a sense of humor is to "discover the elf in yourself." He recommends tapping our inner resources when searching for humor. This includes identifying times we can laugh at ourselves by finding that which is humorous in even difficult or embarrassing situations. Even life's most embarrassing moments can be funny with the passage of time. As Goodman wrote: "Holding a mirror to ourselves and our reality is one of the best ways of taking ourselves less seriously and of playing with situations rather than getting stuck in them" (p. 10). Charles Kuralt in his book *A Life on the Road* tells a story about Marlon Brando which shows the need for finding humor in ourselves. Kuralt was in Olympia, Washington to cover a disagreement between the state of Washington and the Puyallup Indians. The Indians believed they had the right to fish for salmon at any time, including out of season, as long as they were on the reservation. The state disagreed. Brando showed up on the scene to lend his support to the Indian's cause. Brando's purpose, as described by Kuralt, was to "catch an illegal salmon on reservation waters, get arrested, and make headlines to publicize the Indian cause." Unfortunately, Brando was not a very good fisherman. He went out on several mornings and "trolled a salmon lure from a boat with a flotilla of photographers following and the Fish and Game officers watching from a respectful distance.'' No matter how hard he tried Brando could not catch a fish. He tried from "mid-morning until late afternoon, in bright sun and driving rain, but the salmon would not yield to his fame.'' One day he did find a dead salmon in the water. However, "He presented this deceased relic to the officers triumphantly, expecting to be arrested at last. The chief of the detail regarded the limp fish suspiciously, sniffed it and handed it back.'' Brando's fishing expedition ended with the entire incident a joke to everyone except him. Clearly, Marlon Brando would have benefited from finding the humor in this situation.

Another technique Goodman recommends for finding humor within us is developing our personal Murphy's Law. For example, here is a Murphy's Law list for one parent:

1. The later he or she is for school, the more knots in your child's shoelace.
2. The closer you are to the family vacation trip, the more likely one of the children will get sick.
3. The longer the trip the sooner you hear "are we almost there?"
4. Someone will have to use the bathroom within five minutes of passing a rest stop.
5. A child's desire for a toy is directly proportional to the number of times it is seen on a television commercial.
5a. (A corollary to 5) The more a child wants a toy the quicker it becomes boring.
6. The more often you tell a child to do something, the less likely he or she is to do it.
7. The bigger the audience, the worse the behavior.

Similar lists could be developed for activity directors as well as for residents.

Get with it. Goodman's third rule is to "get with it." He explains that we can either laugh at someone or with someone. In the first instance, laughter can be harmful. It is typified by humor based on contempt, abuse, sarcasm, and an exclusive approach. Laughing at people causes divisions. On the other hand, laughing with someone is based on empathy, caring, and an inclusive approach. It creates positive bonds. Goodman sees a need for sensitivity in humor. As he states: "Humor is laughter made from pain–not pain inflicted by laughter."

Practice the 5 Ps. The fourth guideline detailed by Goodman is to follow the rule of the 5 Ps. They are: practice, practice, practice, practice, practice. He recommends procedures, such as observing professional comics and their techniques, which will help develop a humor sense. He identifies a variety of skills and techniques, including exaggeration, understatement, mirroring reality, juxtaposition, reversals, word play, and creating new ideas, as effective humor enhancers. We would add incongruence to this list. Goodman provides detailed descriptions of these methods, as well as ways to incorporate them into programs. Some of his techniques for practicing are included below.

Johnny Carson has built his career at least partly on exaggeration. His statements, such as "Boy, it was so (whatever) today" are then followed by a reaction from the audience: "How (whatever) was it?" to which Carson will provide the exaggeration. Comedian Joey Adams (1968) stated that "all you need is the word *that*, a little imagination and a lot of exaggeration" to create humor. Some examples from Adams include:

She was so rich that she bathed in a solid gold tub and left a 14 carat ring

He was so nervous that he kept coffee awake

He had such a big mouth he could eat a banana sideways.

An activity designed to answer the question How _____ was it? will provide an opportunity for comic relief. (Further hints for incorporating humor into a program are provided later in this chapter.)

Mirroring reality involves viewing everyday events and finding the humor in them. We live in a funny world and all it takes is keeping our eyes open. For example, as I am working on this there is a report on the evening news about a summer camp for dogs. Dogs and owners go away to camp for a week and do traditional camp activities at a cost of several hundred dollars! Goodman cites the work of Erma Bombeck and Candid Camera as two examples of humor resulting from holding a mirror to reality. Looking at reality through humorous eyes can take some of the sting out of life. Bennett Cerf (1972), in a book with the intriguing title, *Stories to Make You Feel Better*, provides a variety of stories of people who looked at reality with a humorous eye. For example:

> A Purdue graduate returned home from his twenty-fifth class reunion in a very chastened mood. "My classmates," he told his wife sadly, "have all gotten so fat and bald they didn't recognize me."

> The late Henry L. Mencken evolved a happy formula for answering all controversial letters. He simply replied, "Dear Sir (or Madam): You may be right."

Since it is not possible to reiterate all he wrote, it is recommended readers read Goodman's work. (A reference for *Laughing Matters* is provided later in this chapter. Additional materials and information may be ordered at the same address.) The HUMOR Project can be a major source of ideas for personal and professional humor development.

Humor: A Tonic You Can Afford

The above title is from the book by Ewers et al. (1983) describing a demonstration project initiated by the Andrus Volunteers (a group of older adults) at Saint John of God Nursing Hospital and Residence in Los Angeles. The project was called "Life Enrichment Through Humor In Long-Term Care Facilities." The program initially included 14 residents of the facility, although over the course of the project 60 of the 77 residents eventually participated. The results of the program are described in Chapter II. The actual program will be delineated here.

The program started with the premise that humor is "a disposition of mind or feeling to make life more tolerable and enjoyable, ranging all the way from pleasant feelings and spontaneous enjoyment to "belly laughs." The program was scheduled for approximately one hour per week and included a variety of activities. The objectives of the humor intervention were to (1) revive and activate a sense of humor in residents, (2) develop activities which were primarily humorous in content, (3) involve residents emotionally, mentally and physically in the program.

The initial step in the program was the development of sufficient resources and materials for a six week program. Resources such as clubs, groups, recreation departments, colleges, calendars of special events, and a variety of humorous books are some of the resources gathered. The process of "filling your humor toolbox" is essential to program success. The actual program included a wide spectrum of activities:

1. Sing-Alongs using familiar tunes were one program component.

2. Old films were also used as part of the program. The project relied on films from public libraries as well as from museums and colleges. Films which elicited reminiscence, amusing observations and discussion were selected.

3. Melodrama using poems or dramas with exaggerated conflicts, emotion, or plot were used in the program. Alfred Noyes' "The Highwayman" is given as an example. The authors recommend there be an interpretative reader and participants to pantomine, in an exaggerated fashion, the roles in the poem or play. Sound effects, as well as appropriate "boos" and "ahs," can be provided by the audience.

4. Puppet shows were identified as a source of amusement and spontaneity. Paper bag puppets can be constructed as needed.

5. Clothing and accessories representing various countries, or eras, were used in a fashion show.

6. Mementos from recent or past events were useful in developing "Down Memory Lane" events. A "This is Your Life" segment could be incorporated into the program.

7. A rhythm band, combining opportunities for rhythm, music appreciation, and harmony, was incorporated into the program.

8. A variety of parties and celebrations were used on special occasions. National Smile Week and April Fool's Day were celebrated.

In addition to these eight programs, the authors identify a variety of other items in their "Humor Toolbox." Their advice is to "try them."

1. Humor Corner–Include jokes, cartoons, funny articles, tapes, and stories. Residents can contribute to the collection.
2. Bulletin Board–A montage of jokes, one-liners, cartoons and posters which should be periodically changed. Materials removed from the board can be placed in the Humor Corner.
3. Cartoons and one-liners–Cut-out cartoons, jokes, etc., mount on colored paper and place on tables and trays at mealtime and special events.
4. Improvisations–Spontaneously act out situations suggested by residents.
5. Grandma's Attic–Put together a box containing a variety of clothing, towels, old kitchen utensils, sugar bowls, flat irons and other articles from the past. One item can be featured on the bulletin board every week.
6. Presentation of honors–Focus on one resident on a special day, for example a birthday, and prepare a "This is Your Life" program.
7. Storytelling–Find a local storyteller, or a resident with the special talent to tell stories. The library can provide stories to read or tell.
8. What If Session–Ask resident to brainstorm answers to a what if question. Ewers et al. suggest questions such as "What if you could arrange your window, what view would you choose?"
9. Droodles–Droodles are drawings which don't make any sense until given a title. Local bookstores will have books of droodles to use in a program.
10. Daffynitions–A daffynition is a silly definition of a word. Ewers et al. give the following examples:

> Deceit–The place you sit.
> Dieting–Triumph of mind over platter.
> Ducky–The wife of a duke.

Adams (1968) adds the following:

Cargo–What gasoline makes.
TV–Watching machine.
Bathing Beauty–A girl worth wading for.

11. Puns–Have residents create and share puns.
12. Hat Rhythm–After collecting a bunch of old hats, have the residents sit in a circle. As music plays have residents take hold of their neighbor's hat on the count of 1 and on the count of 2 put on their neighbor's hat. This continues until all players have worn each hat. The authors recommend having a Polaroid camera available during this activity.

It is recommended that the book *Humor: The Tonic You Can Afford* be added to any humor resource list. The information provided above is only a small part of the useful material in this publication.

Allen Klein and the Healing Power of Humor

In his book entitled *The Healing Power of Humor: Techniques for Getting Through Loss, Setbacks, Upsets, Disappointments, Difficulties, Trial, Tribulations, and All That Not-So-Funny Stuff* (1989), Klein provides 14 techniques for adding humor to life. He identifies these 14 techniques as part of a daily dose of Vitamin H (Humor). In addition to discussing each technique, Klein provides "Learn-To-Laugh Exercises" which will be a valuable addition to anyone's humor toolbox.

1. Klein recommends being prepared for life's difficult moments by anticipating them and having a humorous response. For example, he tells of one person who carries a Get Out of Jail Free card for use when stopped by a police officer. He recommends using the line, "For an encore ladies and gentlemen, I will now . . ." when experiencing unexpected events such as spilling coffee, locking keys in cars and dropping groceries. An activity designed to develop one-liners to use when life's unexpected problems arise would be a good addition to a humor program.

2. Klein suggests using humor to diffuse a difficult situation or to turn difficult situations into humorous ones. One of the authors subscribed to a running magazine after reading of a special offer to mail new subscribers a training log. The training log never arrived and the subscription went unpaid. After several letters from the publisher asking for payment, one arrived expressing their regret the bill had not been paid. The letter included phrases such as "in order to restore your credit with us . . . ," "we assume this was an oversight and this letter will result in your payment being sent," "please pay promptly so you will receive our next issue," and "if you have already sent payment, please disregard this letter." This letter earned a response expressing regret the log had not been received. The letter was addressed directly to the subscription manager with parallel phrases such as "in order to restore your credibility with me . . . ," "please respond promptly so you will receive your check," and "If you have already sent the log, please disregard this letter." Not only did the letter turn the situation into a humorous one, it also resulted in delivery of not one, but two training logs.

Klein suggests structuring an exercise around developing "I have bad news and good news for you" scenarios in order to find humor in bad situations. For example, "the bad news is the price of haircuts is going up. The good news is you are going bald."

3. Klein also values using exaggeration to make difficult times less painful. He suggests exaggerating feelings until they become so absurd you laugh at yourself and your situation.

4. Klein defines irony as getting the exact opposite of what you expect. He suggests finding irony by looking at the relationship of how things started to how they ended up. Ask residents to share incidents in their lives where the way things concluded was not congruent with what was expected. Examples might include blind dates, new purchases, family matters, religious experiences, job related events, or moving into a long term care facility.

5. There is a need to approach life with a positive attitude. Klein tells a story of a woman he would meet every day while they were both walking their dogs. She would always report on the latest crime news from the neighborhood. After several months of hearing about rapes, robberies and fires from the woman, the "Voice of

Doom'' as he called her, Klein realized he could cross the street, walk his dog in the opposite direction, and avoid the woman. He believes we all have the opportunity to ''cross the street'' by adopting a positive outlook on life. The way we view things depends on our attitude. One of several attitude enhancing activities Klein recommends is keeping a ''joy journal'' listing positive events and gifts that are experienced every day. It would include anything valued for its contribution to life. A good meal, a warm smile, an unexpected visitor, or a pleasurable activity may become part of a resident's joy journal. He also suggests drawing a picture, or getting a photo, of yourself laughing and posting this in a prominent place as a reminder you *can* laugh. Attaching such a picture to the door of a resident's room may provide needed affirmation that laughter is still possible.

6. The incorporation of humorous props into a long term care facility will help create a humor environment. The Humor Bulletin Board and the Humor Corner are examples of such environmental manipulation. Klein recommends bubbles for blowing as a prop. Groucho Marx glasses are a commonly used prop, as are red clown noses. Toys and animals may also serve as humor props. Residents can be asked to identify props which they view as humorous, or stress reducing, and these could be introduced into the long term care facility.

7. Klein believes smiling, whether real or forced, can make a person feel better. It provides both a physical and a psychological boost. If that is the case, residents should be encouraged to smile, smile, smile. Possibly every activity should be started with one minute of smiling.

8. Child's play is spontaneous and unencumbered by convention or rules. Klein recommends taking a fresh, playful, look at life. Look at crises with a fresh perspective and maybe things will not be so bad. This involves being open to ideas and looking at things with what Klein calls the ''beginner's mind.''

9. A certain amount of silliness may be therapeutic. For example, writing down the name of everyone who has angered you all week may be helpful. However, it may be more helpful, as Klein suggests, to write them down on a piece of toilet paper and flush them down the toilet. He also suggests listing all the obscenities you

know and giving each a number. Whenever you get upset, select three numbers and shout them out. Nonsense provides an escape from the structure and order of life and may be particularly beneficial to residents of long term care facilities. The serious world of a nursing home demands some non-serious episodes and events. One activity director periodically comes to work in a clown outfit or some similar nonsensical garb.

10. Words are labels which give meaning to objects. Renaming objects has the potential to change attitudes toward them. Klein recommends renaming experiences and objects which are disturbing. For example, nicknaming people who disturb you can result in humor being introduced into the situation. Klein discusses a long term care facility where rewording was used to describe abilities of residents. Residents who must use wheelchairs or walkers to get around are differentiated from those not in need of such assistance by the terms CANE and ABLE. A similar rewording process using words often encountered in long term care facilities could be used as part of a humor program.

11. There is a need to let go of problems and accept what life brings. Rather than being frustrated with things which can't be changed, individuals should learn to accept them. Ask residents to list all the things which are bothering them. Identify the ones which can be changed and put the others on what Klein calls a "forget-it-list" or, as he suggests, attach them to a helium balloon and let them go.

12. There is a need to laugh at ourselves. Laughing at our own foibles, disabilities, or quirks not only makes them less disturbing but also prevents others from feeling uncomfortable with them. Asking residents to share their most embarrassing moment, if they are comfortable doing so, will result in a great deal of laughter, as well as empathy.

13. Residents in long term care facilities can certainly identify the disadvantages in their lives. Finding the positive aspects of residency may help residents. Klein quotes a Zen poem that illustrates this point, "Since my house burned down, I now have a better view of the rising moon." It may be difficult to see the rising moon in a long term care facility, but Klein does provide activities which may help to identify the positive aspects of life.

14. Klein mirrors the opinion of several individuals cited in this volume who believe that humor is everywhere. Even the most difficult of environments and situations can include humor if individuals are open to it. Books, magazines, movies, television, cartoons, and other people can all provide humor.

Klein's book is an invaluable resource for developing humor programs. It provides specific and useful suggestions which will help professionally as well as personally in using humor in daily life.

FACILITATING HUMOR

Permission to Laugh

Case 1

I received a referral noting that Mrs. Luther, age 65, was exceedingly distressed while undergoing her first 2 kidney dialysis procedures. Our intervention was requested to reduce the stress of subsequent experiences.

This therapist encountered Mrs. Luther as she began her third dialysis procedure. The patient appeared teary-eyed and extremely tense. I talked reassuringly with Mrs. Luther and explained our program's interventions to reduce tension during the dialysis procedure. I engaged two veteran dialysis patients in a quiz activity and invited Mrs. Luther to join us. Although she noted that the quiz involved several of her favorite TV programs she quickly added that she was "too ill" to participate at that time. Mrs. Luther closely followed the progress of the game but took none of the opportunities to participate.

Before leaving the unit, Dr. Amsel and Nurse Cafferty paused near the activity. They started a great row regarding this year's Emmy nominees, gave the wrong answers to several quiz questions, and took a minute to laugh and kibitz with participants. Mrs. Luther, who volunteered the correct information to supplant Dr. Amsel's errors, continued to participate long after the staff left the unit. She was eagerly awaiting us upon our next visit.

There are certain situations in life in which we perceive that laughter is virtually forbidden. Certainly Mrs. Luther did not consider the dialysis unit as a place to go for a good time. The imposing devices of high technology, the sterile severity of the environment, the purposeful activity of highly trained professionals sharing their expertise in hushed tones all served to reinforce Mrs. Luther's notion that this was a place to suffer, not to chuckle. If a humor program is to achieve the desired outcomes, patients must feel that it is OK to laugh, indeed that it is good to laugh.

When is it inappropriate for a patient to laugh in a treatment setting? –whenever the patient doesn't want to. The hospital experience gives rise to a variety of intensely felt emotions and there should be safe outlets for expressing all of them. Humor is not an emotion but rather a vehicle for expressing emotions. These feelings may be as disparate as joy, anger, and love. The message that we are trying to convey is not that you must laugh but rather that it is OK to laugh. We don't wish to impose humor but we do want to make it a viable option.

Laughter Inhibitors

Our primary task in setting the stage for humor programs is removal of the prohibitions against laughing. Laughter inhibitors arise from three sources: from the physical environment, from the human environment, and from the patient.

The Physical Environment. In the last decade, institutions have made some radical changes in the appearances of facility interiors. The development of new materials capable of withstanding rigorous cleaning have given designers more options. Competition among health care providers has, in many cases, injected the impetus to effect improvements. Still, there remain institutions in which the ambience screams "tighten up" rather than "lighten up." Humorous activities have difficulty achieving their potentials in heavy environments. A good place to start a humor program, therefore, is with an inspection of the facility. Is the environment totally predictable or is there a place for a porch swing, a puzzling antique gismo, or a *trompe l'oeil* picture? Are there comedy corners or other spaces for framed cartoons and jokes that can be readily changed? Are framed cartoons available for residents to select for display in their rooms? Cartoons get stale after first-reading but their message that it's-OK-to-laugh-in-this-room remains vital.

Treatment rooms and offices may also be done in early American humor. Several years ago, two of my former graduate students sent me a wedding picture. It was the standard, professional wedding photograph of the bride and groom with one addition to the traditional raiment. The demure couple was wearing Groucho Marx glasses, big noses, bushy eyebrows, mustaches and all. After falling over laughing, I gave the framed picture a prominent position on my bookcase. Several days later a distraught student came to my office, certain that a scheduling glitch had added years to her college sentence. With much hand-wringing she began to explain her catastrophe. Suddenly she stopped midsentence and, staring agape at the picture, blurted, "Oh my gosh, is that for real?" We both laughed and shared our admiration for the couple's ability to keep their senses of humor at such a moment. When the student returned to her problem she appeared more relaxed and, I think, gratified to know that she was dealing with a "real" person. Although I have acquired more recent photos of my friends, "the picture" remains above my desk where it continues to help me and my students keep our perspectives in times of stress.

The Human Environment. A phenomenon known to people working in health care is that different units of the same hospital, even units serving similar diagnostic groups, can exude very different atmospheres. Some wards greet you with a colorful poster, gentle sounds from a volunteer classical guitar player, or the wagging tail of a clean puppy. Other wards resist any departure from traditional solemnity. It is not the objective of a humor program to transform all personnel into comedians. It is important, however, that staff understand the potential benefits of the program and support its activities wherever they are consistent with quality care-giving practices.

Staff resistance to raising the humor quotient can result from adherence to two beliefs: (1) the fear that laughter undermines control, and (2) the belief that important people don't kid around.

Laughter and Control. Free laughter flows from a free spirit and is indeed a sign that the individual has not ceded all control to others. Laughter drains the power from fear. Laughter pierces inflated posturing. Because of these principles, laughter will work to subvert coercive authority. Tyrants are, therefore, fairly humorless figures except in the use of ridicule.

The humor that is shared with another, however, can be very affirming. Humor indicates inclusion rather than exclusion. Humor can also communicate respect and caring. Humor is a means of bonding among people and has been shown to reduce the perceived distance between people. The leader who is attempting to foster understanding and gain cooperation will find humor to be an asset.

Laughter and Respect. Although we have come a long way from our Puritan heritage, many adults, at some level of consciousness, still associate laughter with frivolity, triviality, and childishness. A serious demeanor is attached to maturity, power, and success. For this type of person, working in a solemn setting, performing solemn tasks affirms their perception of their importance. The humor program does not.

Studies of the use of humor in small groups indicate that humorous exchanges are more frequently initiated by members of higher status. In health care settings, staff acquire status concomitant to their power and expertise. Patients may wait for staff to initiate humor or they may tentatively test the waters to assess others' response. If humor threatens the self-images of unit staff, the ward could be a cheerless place.

Patient Attitudes. Patients may also embrace attitudes that defeat humor. The belief that this setting is too serious to laugh in, that people will be offended, is a certain laugh squelcher. Perhaps George Bernard Shaw most eloquently advocated for humor amid serious times and places when he stated, "Life does not cease to be funny when people die, any more than it ceases to be serious when people laugh."

Sometimes we encounter an angry patient who protests that he is already humiliated by disability and that he is not going to endure the further indignity of being silly. Oddly enough, humor has been the vehicle that has enabled many to maintain their dignity despite the insults of disability. Our angry patients may benefit from viewing some role models or discussing how persons like Franklin Roosevelt used humor to prevail over disability.

Another threat to humor is the patient's concern that if he laughs no one will know that he is hurting. With the high cost of health care, the least a patient can do is look sickly. If there are no contra-indications, we need to affirm again and again that it is good to laugh. Some physicians have gone so far as issuing prescriptions to patients, writing orders to laugh. It may also be helpful to acknowledge our patients' courage to laugh in spite of fear and pain.

Humor Inventories

Admitting humor into our communications with patients requires sensitivity. We can elicit conversation from the patient and try to ascertain where the client is emotionally before interjecting humor or we can throw out a gently humorous greeting and assess its reception. Sensitivity requires effort and even with our best effort we sometimes misread the situation and go in with a zinger that results in the patient feeling that we've trivialized his problem. The occasion calls for an immediate apology and a reconsideration of the topic with our most intense affect. It does not merit a renouncing of humor and the adoption of a fail-safe, humorless demeanor.

If care givers and receivers could identify their own attitudes and beliefs regarding humor, they could decide which attitudes were blocking their effective uses of humor and which attitudes and skills they wished to nurture. The following exercises are offered to structure explorations of our humorous natures. The activities are designed to stimulate small group discussion or individual contemplation about the development of individual humor styles, about our personal tastes in humor, and about attitudes, values, and behaviors that we wish to reaffirm or reject. The questions may generate humorous as well as unpleasant recollections. If childhoods were bereft of humor it might be more difficult to fully enjoy humor today. More fun can be found in life, however, and later activities will help clients to develop, alter, or rediscover their senses of humor.

Since some of the assessment instruments reveal personal preferences for types of humor, the information gleaned may be used for planning future activities and for collecting humorous materials for individual patients.

WHAT'S SO FUNNY

Where did we get our ideas and behaviors regarding humor? Some of them were probably adopted from the things we saw and heard when we were children. Identify some people who influenced you when you were a child. Four figures are suggested below, but you may replace them with others. Check the items that most apply to each person.

favorite elementary school teacher _____
   mother
      father
         most feared person _____
            other _____

__ __ __ __ __ A. laughed a lot
__ __ __ __ __ B. laughed sometimes
__ __ __ __ __ C. almost never laughed

__ __ __ __ __ A. was often playful
__ __ __ __ __ B. was sometimes playful
__ __ __ __ __ C. was never playful

__ __ __ __ __ A. laughed at me a lot
__ __ __ __ __ B. Laughed at me some
__ __ __ __ __ C. almost never laughed at me

__ __ __ __ __ A. told me/us jokes
__ __ __ __ __ B. told me/us funny incidents from his/her past
__ __ __ __ __ C. did funny antics
__ __ __ __ __ D. read or told us funny stories
__ __ __ __ __ E. read us the comics
__ __ __ __ __ F. found a lot of humor in daily life
__ __ __ __ __ G. played pranks on us or others
__ __ __ __ __ H. laughed only, or mostly, when drinking alcohol

Who did you laugh the most with when you were a child? _____

Circle one: I laugh **more than, about the same as, less than** my mother did when she was my age.

I laugh **more than, about the same as, less than** my father did.

WHERE DID YOU GET THAT FUNNY IDEA?

What messages about humor were conveyed to you when you were a child? By their words or behaviors, who imparted those messages?

_____Laughing at people shows superiority.

      conveyed by_____

_____Sharing laughter is a form of caring.

_____Laughing is embarrassing.

_____Having fun is what life is all about.

_____Laughter indicates that you are not earnest about the situation.

_____Your laughter indicates that you don't respect me.

_____Your laughter is an attempt to subvert my authority.

_____Interject laughter frequently while trying to make a point. This will indicate that you're not competitive nor a threat to your opponent.

_____Laughter decreases the distance between us.

_____Laughing at someone is hurtful and diminishes the person laughing.

_____Life is fun.

_____If you're having fun, you're not working hard enough.

_____Laughter makes a scary situation less fearsome.

_____

_____Laughter is an acceptable replacement for crying.

_____

_____Women should laugh to indicate that their opinions are not put forth as credible options.

_____

_____Life is pretty funny.

_____

_____Laughter can be unconstrained while drinking, but should otherwise be held in check by responsible adults.

_____

_____Your laughter in my presence is a mockery of the success and power that I have achieved.

_____

other messages:

Circle the messages that you feel are true for you today.
Place a star in front of the messages that your behaviors send to others today.

_____

FUNNY PLACES

Places where it was *not* OK to laugh when I was a child:

___ in church
___ in school
___ in _____ class
        teacher's name
___ at the doctor's office
___ at _____ house
        friend or relative's
___ at the dinner table
___ in _____ presence
           name
___ other _____

When you were a child, where did you laugh the most?_____

What places today do you find it inappropriate or difficult to laugh in? _____

In your travels, in which places did you encounter people with the best senses of humor?_____

Where did you encounter the worst senses of humor? _____

What does my room or office reflect about my sense of humor?

Does my room or office make people feel that it's OK to laugh there?

Draw a rough floor plan of the house you lived in when you were a child. Label the rooms. In which room did you have the most fun?_____

In which room did you have the least fun?_____

Identify a funny incident that happened in each room.

SPEAKING OF HUMOR

Rate these quotations by giving 3 stars to those you think are sensational, two stars if they're pretty good, and one star if they're OK. Circle the quotes you disagree with.

1. The one serious conviction that a man should have is that nothing is to be taken too seriously (Samuel Butler).
2. There is no cure for birth or death save to enjoy the interval (George Santayana).
3. Life does not cease to be funny when people die, any more than it ceases to be serious when people laugh (George Bernard Shaw).
4. The best doctors in the world are doctor diet, doctor quiet, and doctor merryman (Jonathan Swift).
5. Everything is funny as long as it is happening to someone else (Will Rogers).
6. Laughing is the sensation of feeling good all over and showing it principally in one spot (Josh Billings).
7. Good humor is goodness and wisdom combined (Owen Meredith).

8. You know what happens when you stifle a laugh; it goes straight to your hips (Annette Goodheart).
9. The greatest exercise for the heart is lifting someone up (anon.).
10. He who laughs, lasts (anon.).
11. It is my belief that you cannot deal with the most serious things in the world unless you understand the most amusing (Winston Churchill).
12. The best thing about humor is that it shows people that they're not alone (Sid Caesar).
13. If you can find humor in something, you can survive it (Bill Cosby).
14. Comedy is acting out optimism (Robin Williams).
15. Humor is the great thing, the saving thing after all. The minute it crops up, all our hardnesses yield, all our irritations and resentments slip away, and a sunny spirit takes their place (Mark Twain).
16. You can learn more about a man in an hour of play than in a lifetime of conversation (Plato).
17. Any man who has had the job I've had and didn't have a sense of humor wouldn't still be here (Harry Truman).
18. Comedy is the last refuge of the nonconformist mind (Gilbert Selds).
19. Most folks are about as happy as they make up their minds to be (Abe Lincoln).
20. My sense of humor was vital to my survival in prison. As soon as I started [joking], I immediately felt in control of myself (Anatoly Shcharansky).
21. Buffoons who take themselves seriously are often the funniest of all (David Rossie).
22. We don't laugh because we're happy–we're happy because we laugh (William James).

Questions to ponder:

Was Abe Lincoln right (# 19)? Who's responsibility is it to find some humor each day? How can we find more of it?

Do you agree with Bill Cosby (# 13)? In what tough situations have you used humor or have seen others use humor? Can you recall the humor that was used?

When you laugh about your weaknesses, disabilities, or problems, does it make you feel more in control as it did for Anatoly Shcharansky (# 20)?

CHARTING YOUR SENSE OF HUMOR

I laugh most at (circle one of each trio):

1. Lilly Tomlin	Andrew Dice Clay	Bob Hope
2. Three Stooges	Billy Crystal	Joan Rivers
3. Bill Cosby	Don Rickles	Robin Williams
4. Art Buchwald	Andy Rooney	Louis Grizzard
5. Roseanne Barr	Johnny Carson	Lucille Ball
6. Fred Allen	Mae West	Will Rogers
7. Tracey Ullman	Benny Hill	Margaret Thatcher
8. Whoopi Goldberg	Groucho Marx	Steve Martin
9. Steve Allen	Red Buttons	Jack Benny
10. Red Skelton	Milton Berle	Sid Caesar
11. Betty White	Sophie Tucker	Buddy Hackett
12. Burns & Allen	Abbott & Costello	Marx Bros.
13. Buster Keaton	Charlie Chaplin	W. C. Fields
14. Katzenjammer Kids	Andy Capp	The Far Side

15. My favorite comedian is_____.
16. My favorite cartoon or comic strip is_____.
17. My favorite TV comedy or sitcom is_____.
18. My favorite funny movie is_____.
19. I would rate my sense of humor as (circle one):

    0 1 2 3 4 5 6 7 8 9 10
    awful   fantastic

20. My spouse's sense of humor is:

    0 1 2 3 4 5 6 7 8 9 10
    awful   fantastic

21. My mother's sense of humor:

    0 1 2 3 4 5 6 7 8 9 10
    awful   fantastic

22. My father's sense of humor:
    0 1 2 3 4 5 6 7 8 9 10
    awful   fantastic
23. Circle all the words that apply to your sense of humor.
    Check the words that apply to your mother's humor.
    Star the words that apply to your father's humor.

dry	hilarious	sarcastic	satirical
surprise	mocking	capricious	childish
ridicule	silly	stoic	witty
droll	uproarious	cynical	disdainful
gleeful	slapstick	cerebral	playful
childlike	guarded	uninhibited	teasing
physical	divisive	joyful	flirtatious
dark	scornful	antic	facetious
farcical	raconteur	bizarre	ribald
buffoon	hostile	risque	bumpkin
sardonic	corny	zany	sarcastic
waggish	deadpan	whimsical	smart alec
prankster	off-beat	grotesque	insulting

24. Which 4 words are most descriptive of your humor style?

    _____   _____

    _____   _____

25. Which 4 are least like your humor style?

    _____   _____

    _____   _____

26. Words associated with my laugh are (circle):

gusty	nervous	melodious	tentative
raucous	spontaneous	giggly	embarrassing
uncontrolled	suppressed	polite	sneezy
snorty	harumph	harsh	piercing
knee-slapping	chuckling	hooty	unbridled
ho ho ho	tee hee hee	ha ha ha	ha

27. The person who has a laugh I love to hear:

    _____

28. People I have laughed the most with:

    _____

What is it about their laugh or manner that invites you to laugh with them?

A FUNNY THING HAPPENED ON THE WAY...

Chronicle some of the funny things that have happened in your life. If items on this sheet bring recollections of humorous incidents, you may note them below or compile them in a journal.

Funny things that happened when I:

1. was in grade school
2. was in high school
3. learned to drive
4. got my first car
5. played sports
6. got married
7. was in church
8. was in the military
9. had a pet
10. went to camp
11. went on vacation
12. tried to cook
13. first tried to smoke
14. got my first job
15. was doing chores

Funny things that happened:

16. at Christmas
17. in my home town
18. at Halloween
19. to my friends and me
20. to my brothers and/or sisters and me
21. to my mother
22. to my father
23. to my grandparents
24. My most embarrassing moment occurred when:
25. Boy, did I get in trouble when:

26. Oh, did I have a mess when:
27. I got to giggling so hard when:
28. The funniest prank I ever saw was:

HUMOR TECHNIQUES YOU CAN USE

Opportunities to Involve Staff

When administrators and clinical personnel can model healthy humor behaviors it not only gives patients or residents permission to laugh but it provides a catalyst for the humor program. The following activities provide opportunities for staff who are willing and able to share some therapeutic humor with patients.

1. The Joke Board–The first thing every good humor program needs is a renewable supply of jokes and cartoons. As soon as patients and volunteers have clipped a good supply of material, deliver the jokes to one or two consenting staff members and ask them to select their 10 favorite jokes or cartoons. They may also draw from their own sources of favorite jokes. The humor is then posted on the joke board along with the names of the week's featured humor selectors. As the board draws interest, patients are included among the featured selectors.

2. Name that Comedian–Provide some game personnel and residents with joke material and ask them to prepare a joke for audio-taping. Extract segments from recorded comic material of Jack Benny, Fred Allen, Bob Hope et al., and intersperse your composite recording with jokes by your house comedians. Use the quiz for group activities or check it out to individuals for their listening pleasure.

3. Humor Photos–Snap close-up photos of patient/staff duos (or singles) holding humorous big signs like, "Grin & Ignore It!" Post the pictures around the facility in surprising places.

4. The House Laugh Track–It's not nearly as much fun to laugh by yourself as it is to join along with twenty hardy laughers. In fact, since laughter is so contagious, no program should be without a recorded laugh track. A hilarious commercial tape is available that features psychotherapist, Annette Goodheart, and physician, Steve

Allen, Jr. (see "Resources" at the end of this unit). You can add local staff and resident laughers to this track or make a track of your own. If you're starting from scratch, you'll need a nucleus of uninhibited laughers to get the group rolling. Once completed, you can use the track as a quiz to identify local laughs, as an activity background to set a merry atmosphere, or as a focus for explorations on the theme of variety-in-laugh-styles-and-the-joy-of-owning-your-own.

5. Photo Captions–Creating humorous captions to accompany newspaper clippings is a reliable activity for generating humor. President Reagan, or his writer, was adept with this medium. At a meeting of the Washington Press Club, a slide was projected that depicted the President picking up a telephone as he and Mikhail Gorbachev looked at their watches. The President narrated, "When Gorbachev visits, I try to let him experience life in America. Here, I'm telling him, 'This is the way it works, if they don't get here within half an hour, we get the pizza free.'"

A local variation of this design adds even more fun. Take black and white photographs of staff and residents as they interact around the house. You may take candid shots as people go about their usual tasks or you may conspire with people to create poses indicative of action. After you have selected the photographs that are ripe for captioning, explain your intentions to the people in the pictures and secure their permissions to use the photographs. Affix cartoon balloons to the photos where needed and duplicate them with a copying machine. Distribute to residents and staff to complete the cartoon balloons with whatever words they deem most fun. For more fun, post the humor art around the facility.

Activities for Humor Generation

1. The Humor File–From a large central collection of jokes and cartoons, residents are encouraged to select their favorites and file them in a folder or large envelope. Residents keep their files for review and expansion. If used as a group activity, participants can share their number one favorites at the close of the search.

2. The Joke of the Week–Residents submit their favorite joke for

the week. It may have been a funny story they read of a joke told by their grandchild or other visitor. To encourage visitor participation in the humor program, this activity can be modified to Visitors' Joke of the Week. Select the winning entries and post them on the humor board.

3. The Joke Swap–At the weekly appointed hour, residents meet to exchange jokes and humorous anecdotes. Residents may bring their humor files noting their recent acquisitions.

4. Humor Journals–For clients who enjoy writing, humor journaling may double their pleasure. Journals can be used to record funny incidents that are part of the family history. These journals and their contents are sure to be treasured by other family members. Journals can also be used to increase awareness of the humor that surrounds us on a daily basis. It may be helpful to provide journalists with a brief list of questions to stimulate inquiry:

1. What was the funniest thing that happened today or this week?
2. What was the most humorous thing I saw?
3. What was the most humorous thing someone said?
4. What humorous item did I read?
5. What was the funniest thing I saw on TV?

As writers become more aware of good humor material, they will keep their journals handy for quick notations of humorous incidents. Residents may take their journals to the Joke Swaps or submit material to the house newsletter.

5. Absurd Exaggerations–There are many devices of logic and language that comedians use to create humor. Clients who are interested in expanding their own skills at creating humor will find some practical tips from the books of Steve Allen (1987) and Allen Klein (1989). A common device is to exaggerate a description and stretch it to colorful and absurd limits. The following challenge allows participants to try their hands at creating this type of humor.

HOW BAD WAS IT?

1. That Bingo caller was so slow!
   How slow was he?
   He was so slow that _____
2. That doctor is so charming! _____
3. Those biscuits are so heavy! _____
4. That dog was so ugly! _____
5. That stethoscope is so cold! _____
6. That bird feeder draws so many birds! _____
7. I had to wait for _____ for so long! _____
8. It rained so hard! _____
9. That pill is so big! _____
10. That movie was so funny! _____
11. I was so hungry! _____
12. Our town was so small! _____

6. Clowning–Clowns grant instant permission to enjoy nonsense and silliness. It's always safe to laugh with a clown. Some facilities have established a clown referral service whereby visitors can stop by or call the reception desk and order a clown for their friend or relative. When the volunteer clown arrives at the agency, he or she visits the referred patients or residents, bringing cheer and a message from the visitors who referred him. In many cities, teams of volunteer clowns are available to visit health care centers, clown around, and even to paint staff and patients in clownface.

7. Comedy Video–Have everyone in the group choose a favorite joke and practice telling it for a week. Video record your jokesters and make the comedy tape available to bed patients. Feature a special viewing for dinner entertainment.

Short Subjects

Sometimes a fleeting moment of humor is all that is needed to break a gloomy mood and lighten the atmosphere. Some of these ideas, or modifications thereof, may be helpful at your facility.

1. Make an entrance in your Groucho Marx nose.
2. Declare Groucho Marx Day on the unit and pass out noses all around.
3. Do your Groucho routine and invite your group to "Walk this way." Give an award to the best Groucho.
4. When reclaiming a noisy group, get their attention with unusual voice inflections.
5. Wear a funny button.
6. Give that shy, sad guy your funny button.
7. Put a silly portrait on your desk or wall.
8. Reserve a conference room and set up a candlelight luncheon for your staff or for a colleague's birthday.
9. Compose some humorous memos for timely distribution.
10. Carry a wind-up toy in your pocket.
11. Have a funny hat day.
12. Create a humor emergency kit: a couple of good jokes, cartoons, a clown nose, a wind-up toy, whatever. Label appropriately and keep it on hand to present to clients or staff who are having a tough day.
13. Take a polaroid picture of the emergency kit recipient in her clown nose.
14. Leave a flower on someone's desk.
15. Leave some silly putty on someone's desk.
16. Post pet pictures. Guess which pet belongs to whom.
17. Have everyone fantasize about winning the lottery.
18. Tell someone how their laugh cheers you up.
19. Design humorous greeting cards.
20. Make a silly face at your clients. Reward the client who can make a sillier face.
21. Wipe all traces of mirth from your faces. Challenge "it" to draw a smile from the group.
22. Take a humor break: Whose laugh do you like to hear? Picture that person laughing. Hear their laughter in your mind. Take a deep breath and smile.
23. Share some favorite comics and comic book with residents.

HUMOR RESOURCES

In addition to many books and articles listed in the reference section, libraries will have a variety of joke books, books of stories, movies, etc., which can be used in humor programs. Other resources are listed below.

Clown Supplies

162 Gregory Island Road, Hamilton, MA 01982.

Computer Software

"The Humor Processor" invites the user to experience and apply the comedy creating process. Uses a variety of joke formulae (exaggeration, cliche rewrites, funny definition, reversal, misdirection) to generate over 100,000 comedic combinations. Designed for IBM PC's and compatibles. About fifty dollars from Responsive Software, 1901 Tunnel Road, Berkeley, CA 94705.

Laughing Matters

A quarterly publication of jokes and humor program ideas and resources. About $15.00 a year. Available from The Humor Project, Subscriptions Department, 110 Spring Street, Saratoga Springs, NY 12866.

Laugh Track

An audiotape featuring the hilarious laughter of Annette Goodheart and Steve Allen, Jr. About $14.00 from Dan and Julie Allen, 104 Greenridge Drive, Horseheads, NY 18485.

American Association for Therapeutic Humor

Produces a newsletter to share information among professionals applying humor in their work. 1441 Shermer Avenue, Suite 110, Northbrook, IL 60062.

The Whole Mirth Catalog

A catalog of humor items. 1034 Page Street, San Francisco, CA 94117.

Creating a Comedy Cart

A guide for creating a lending program of multimedia humor resources. Morton Plant Hospital, 323 Jeffords Street, Clearwater, FL 34617.

Appendix A

Films Shown During the Clemson Humor Project

HUMOR GROUP	SERIOUS GROUP
I Love Lucy	Casablanca
Laurel and Hardy	Wuthering Heights
Amos and Andy	An American in Paris
W.C. Fields	Jezebel
Abbott and Costello	Seven Brides for Seven Brothers
Three Stooges	Westside Story
The Honeymooners	She Wore a Yellow Ribbon
Hold That Ghost	42nd Street
Disorderly Orderly	Little Women
My Favorite Brunette	Goodbye, Mr. Chips
Road to Bali	Cat on a Hot Tin Roof
18 Again	African Queen
Yours, Mine, Ours	High Noon
The Kid	Snows of Kilimanjaro
Breakfast at Tiffany's	A Star is Born
Candid Camera	The Western
Your Show of Shows	Little Princess
At War With the Army	Pygmalion
The Clown	Cocoon
Honey I Shrunk the Kids	Winter People
Mr. Mom	The Robe
Kid With a Broken Halo	ET
Blind Date	The Benny Goodman Story
Mac and Me	Magnificent Obsession
Connecticut Yankee	Johnny Belinda
It's a Wonderful Life	Elmer Gantry
We're No Angels	Mohawk
Young at Heart	Royal Wedding
The Bohemian Girl	On the Waterfront
African Screams	Wicked Stepmother

Return to Mayberry
The Shakiest Gun in the West
Smokey the Bandit
Turner and Hooch
Disorderlies
Pee Wee's Big Adventure
Funny Farm
Going Bananas
The Incredible Mr. Limpet
Uncle Buck
Popeye
Harry and the Hendersons
Charlie Chaplin Films
Little Rascals
Room Service
Stolen Jewels
No Deposit, No Return
Who Framed Roger Rabbit
The Bowery Boys
The Bells of St. Mary's
Animal Crackers
A variety of episodes
of shows such as "I
Love Lucy," "The Three
Stooges," and "Abbott and
Costello" were shown.

Adam's Rib
A Tree Grows in Brooklyn
A Touch of Mink
The Philadelphia Story
Treasure Island
Ten Commandments
Where the Red Fern Grows
To Kill a Mockingbird
Project X
The Boy Who Could Fly
Tale of Two Cities
The Greatest Story Ever Told
Stealing Home
White Christmas
The Natural
High Noon
Love Me Tender
Charade
National Velvet
The Yearling
Mr. Smith Goes to Washington
The Godfather
Hawaii
Let's Get Tough
Dress to Kill
Farewell to Arms
Hush, Hush Sweet Charlotte
Whatever Happened to Baby Jane

REFERENCES

AARP. (1989). *Profiles of Older Americans.* Washington, DC: American Association of Retired Persons.

Abramson, L., Gorber, J., and Seligman, M. (1980). Learned Helplessness in Humans: An Attributional Analysis. In J. Gorber, and M. Seligman (Ed.), *Human Helplessness: Theory and Applications.* New York, NY: Academic Press.

Adams, E. and McGuire, F. (1986). Is Laughter the Best Medicine? A Study of the Effects of Humor on Perceived Pain and Affect. *Activities, Adaptation & Aging, 8* (3-4), 157-175.

Adams, J. (1968). *Joey Adams Encyclopedia of Humor.* New York: Bobbs-Merrill Company.

Allen, S. (1987). *How to be Funny: Discovering the Comic in You.* New York: McGraw-Hill.

Anthony, J., and Benedik, T. (1975). *Depression and Humor Existence.* Boston, MA: Little Brown.

Averill, J. (1969). Anatomic Response Patterns During Sadness and Mirth. *Psychophysiology, 5,* 399-413.

Baltes, M., and Baltes, R. (1986). *The Psychology of Control and Aging.* Hillsdale, NJ: Lawrence, Erlbaum Associates.

Beck, S., and Page, J. (1988). Involvement in Activities and Psychological Well-Being of Retired Men. *Activities, Adaptation & Aging,* 11(1), 31-47.

Berlyne, D. (1972). Humor and Its Kin. In J. Goldstein, and P. McGhee (Ed.), *The Psychology of Humor: Theoretical Perspectives and Empirical Issues.* New York, NY: Academic Press.

Blumenfield, E., and Alpern, L. (1986). *The Smile Connection: How to Use Humor in Dealing with People.* New York, NY: Prentice-Hall, Inc.

Bradburn, N. (1969). *The Structure of Psychological Well-Being.* Chicago, IL: Aldine Publishing Co.

Browning, R. (1979). *Classification and Behavioral Categories of Humor, Wit and Comedy.* Los Angeles, CA: Paper presented at the 2nd International Conference on Humor.

Campbell, D., and Stanley, J. (1963). *Experimental and Quasi-Experimental Designs for Research.* Chicago, IL: Rand McNally College Publishing Co.

Cerf, B. (1972). *Stories to Make You Feel Better.* New York: Random House.

Chapman, A. (1976). Social Aspects of Humorous Laughter, In A. Chapman & H. Foot (Ed.), *Humor and Laughter: Theory, Research and Applications.* London, England: Wiley.

Chapman, A.J. and Foot, H.C. (Eds.) (1977). *It's a Funny Thing, Humor.* Oxford: Pergamon Press.

Christensen, L. (1978). *The Older Person's Experience of Aging: A Psychological*

Study. Unpublished Doctoral Dissertation, California School of Professional Psychology, San Diego.

Cogan, R., Cogan, D., Waltz, W., and McCue, M. (1987). Effects of Laughter and Relaxation on Discomfort Thresholds. *Journal of Behavioral Medicine, 10* (2), 139-143.

Cousins, N. (1979). *Anatomy of an Illness*. New York, NY: Bantam Books.

Crane, A. (1990). Coping through Laughter. *Laugh it Up*, May-June.

Cumming, E., & Henry, W. (1961). *Growing Old: The Process of Disengagement*. New York, NY: Basic Books Int.

Dewey, J. (1894). The Theory of Emotion. *Psychological Review 1*.

Duellman, M., Barris, R, and Kielhofner, G. (1986). Organized Activity and Adaptive Status of Nursing Home Residents. *The American Journal of Occupational Therapy 40*(9), 618-622.

Ewers, M., Jacobson, S., Powers, V., and McConney, P. (1983). *Humor, the Tonic You Can Afford: A Handbook of Ways of Using Humor in Long-term Care*. Los Angeles, CA: Ethel Percy Andrus Gerontological Center.

Fay, R. (1983). *The Defensive Role of Humor in the Management of Stress*. Doctoral Dissertation, United States International University, San Diego, CA.

Freud, S. (1959). Humor. *Collected Papers*. New York, NY: Basic Books.

Freud, S. (1979). *Jokes and their Relation to the Unconscious*. New York, NY: Penguin Books.

Fry, W. (1979). *Catharsis and Arousal: Humor as a Paradigm*. Abstract from an address at the American Psychological Association.

Fry, W. (1982). *The Psychology of Humor*. Salt Lake City, UT: Abstract from an address at the Psychobiology of Health and Healing Conference at Brigham Young University.

Fry, W. (1986). Humor Physiology and the Aging Process. In L. Namehow, K. McCluskey-Fawcett, and P. McGhee (Ed.), *Humor and Aging*. Orlando, FL: Academic Press.

Fry, W., and Allen, M. (1976). Humor as a Creative Experience: The Development of a Hollywood Humorist. In A. Chapman, and H. Foot (Ed.), *Humor and Laughter: Theory, Research and Applications*. London, England: John Wiley & Sons.

Fry, W., and Roder, C. (1969). Humor in a Physiologic Vein. *News on Physiological Instrumentation*, July, 3.

Fry, W., and Roder, C. (1977). The Respiratory Components of Mirthful Laughter. *Journal of Biomedical Society, 19*, 39-50.

Fry, W., and Savin, M. (1982). *Mirthful Laughter and Blood Pressure*. Washington, DC: Paper presented at the 3rd International Conference on Humor.

Fry, W., and Stroft, P. (1971). Mirth and Oxygen Saturation Levels of Peripheral Blood. *Psychotherapy and Psychosomatics, 19*, 76-84.

George, L., and Bearon, L. (1980). *Quality of Life in Older Persons: Meaning and Measurement*. New York, NY: Human Sciences Press.

Goodman, J. (1982). *Laughing Matters: The Magic of Humor in the Workplace, Classroom and Home*. Washington, DC: Paper presented at the 3rd International Conference on Humor.

Goodman, J. (1983). How to Get More Smileage Out of Your Life: Making Sense of Humor, then Serving It. In P. McGhee, and J. Goldstein (Ed.), *Handbook of Humor Research*. New York, NY: Springer-Verlag.

Grotjahn, M. (1957). *Beyond Laughter*. New York, NY: McGraw-Hill Book Co.

Haig, R.A. (1988). *The Anatomy of Humor: Biophychosomal and Therapeutic Perspectives*. Springfield, Illinois: C.C. Thomas.

Havighurst, R. (1972). Lifestyle and Leisure Patterns: Their Evolution through the Life Cycle. *Leisure in Third Age*. Paris, France: International Center for Social Gerontology.

Hobbes, T. (1840). Human Nature. In W. Molesworth (Ed.), *Works*. London, England: Bohn.

Kahana, E., Farchild, T., and Kahana, B. (1982). Adaptation. In D. Mangen, and W. Peterson (Ed.), *Research Instruments in Gerontology*. Minneapolis, MN: University of Minnesota Press.

Kalish, R. (1977). *The Later Years: Social Applications of Gerontology*. Monterey, CC: Brooks/Cole Publishing Co.

Kant, I. (1892). *Kritik of Judgement, Translation J. H. Bernard*. London, England: MacMillan.

Kastenbaum, R., and Sherwood, S. (1972). Viro: A Scale of Assessing Interview Behavior of Elderly People. In D. Kent, R. Kastenbaum, and S. Sherwood (Ed.), *Research Planning and Action for the Elderly: The Power and Potential of Social Science*. New York, NY: Behavioral Publications.

Kelly, J. (undated). *Life in Between: Continuity and Construction*.

Klein, A. (1989). The Healing Power of Humor. *Techniques for Getting Through Loss, Setbacks, Upsets, Disappointment, Difficulties, Trials, Tribulations and all that Not-so-Funny Stuff*. Los Angeles: J. P. Tarcher.

Kuralt, C. (1990). *A Life on the Road*. New York: G. P. Putnam and Sons.

Langer, E. (1983). *The Psychology of Control*. New York, NY: Sage.

Langer, E., and Rodin, J. (1976). The Effects of Choice and Enhanced Responsibility for the Aged: A Field Experiment in an Institutional Setting. *Journal of Personality and Social Psychology*, 34(2), 191-198.

Langevin, R., and Day, H. (1972). Psychological Correlates of Humor. In J. Goldstein, and P. McGhee (Ed.), *The Psychology of Humor: Theoretical Perspectives and Empirical Issues*. New York, NY: Academic Press.

Lawton, M. (1983). Environment and Other Determinants of Well-being in Older People. *The Gerontology*, 23, 349-360.

Lefcourt, H., and Martin, R. (1986). *Humor and Life Stress: Antidote to Adversity*. New York, NY: Springer-Verlag.

Levine, J. (1956). Responses to Humor. *Scientific American*, 194, 31-35.

Levine, J. (1977). Humor as a Form of Therapy: Introduction to Symposium. In A. Chapman, and H. Foot (Ed.), *It's a Funny Thing, Humor*. Oxford, England: Pergamon.

Lorenz, K. (1966). *On Aggression*, translation, M. Wilson. New York, NY: Harcourt, Brace and World.

Ludovici, A. (1933). *The Secret of Laughter*. New York, NY: Viking Press.

Mangen, D. (Nov. 1977). *Non-Random Measurement Error in the Bradburn Affect*

Balance Scale: Toward the Development of a Social Historical Theory of Measurement Error. San Francisco: Paper presented at the 30th annual meeting of the Gerontological Society.

Mannel, R., and McMahon, L. (1982). Humor as Play: Its relationship to Psychological Well-Being during the course of a Day. *Leisure Sciences. 5(2)*, 143-153.

Martin, R., and Lefcourt, H. (1983). Sense of Humor as a Moderator of the Relationship Between Stressors and Moods. *Journal of Personality and Social Psychology, 45*, 1313-1324.

Martineau, W. (1972). A Model of Social Functions of Humor. In J. Goldstein, and P. McGhee (Ed.), *The Psychology of Humor: Theoretical Perspectives and Empirical Issues*. New York, NY: Academic Press.

McDowell, C. (1983). *Leisure Wellness: An Introduction*. Eugene, OR: SunMoon Press.

McGhee, P. (1979). *Humor: Its Origins and Development*. San Francisco, CA: W.H. Freeman and Co.

McGhee, P. (1986). Humor Across the Life Span: Sources of Developmental Change and Individual Differences. In L. Namehow, K.

McGhee, P.E., and Goldstein, J.H. (1983). *Handbook of Humor Research: Volume II Applied Studies*. New York: Springer-Verlag.

Mercer, S., and Kane, R. (1979). Helplessness and Hopelessness Among the Institutionalized Aged: An Experiment. *Health and Social Work*, s(1), 91-116.

Miles, E. (1988). *The Relationship of Sense of Humor to Life Satisfaction, Functional Health, Death Anxiety and Self-Esteem*. Doctoral Dissertation, California School of Professional Psychology, Irvine, CA.

Mindess, H. (1971). *Laughter and Liberation*. Los Angeles, CA: Nash.

Mindess, H., and Turek, J. (1979). *The Study of Humor*. Los Angeles, CA: Antioch University.

Moriwaki, S. (1974). The Affect Balance Scale: A Validity Study with Aged Samples. *Journal of Gerontology, 29,(1)* 73-78.

Morreal, J. (1983). *Taking Laughter Seriously*. Albany, NY: SUNY.

Namehow, L. (1986). Humor as a Database for the Study of Aging. In L. Namehow, K. McCluskey-Fawcett, and P. McGhee (Ed.). *Humor and Aging*, Orlando, FL: Academic Press.

Namehow, L., and Lawton, P. (1976). "Toward an Ecological Theory of Adaptation and Aging." In H. Prokansky, W. Ittleson, and L. Rivlin (Ed.), *Environmental Psychology: People and Their Physical Settings:* New York, NY: Rinehart and Winston.

Napora, J. (1984). "A Study of the Effects of a Program of Humorous Activity of Subjective Well-Being of Senior Adults" Dissertation, University of Maryland, College Park, MD.

Nemeth, P. (1979). *An Investigation into the Relationship Between Humor and Anxiety*. Doctoral Dissertation, United States International University, San Diego, CA.

Neugarten, B. (1974). *Successful Aging: A Conference Report*. Durham, NC: Center for the Study on Aging and Human Development.

Svebac, S. (1975). Respiratory Patterns and Predictors of Laughter. *Psychophysiology, 12*, 62-65.

Tennant, K. (1986). The Effect of Humor on the Recovery Rate of Cataract Patients: A Pilot Study. In L. Namehow, K. McCluskey-Fawcett, and P. McGhee (Ed.), *Humor and Aging*. Orlando, FL: Academic Press.

Vaillant, G. (1977). *Adaptation of Life*. Boston, MA: Little Brown & Co.

Voelkl, J. (1986). Effects of Institutionalization Upon Residents of Extended Care Facilities. *Activities, Adaptation & Aging, 8*(3-4), 37-45.

Walt, K. (1978). Preferred Environments. In S. Kaplan, and R. Kaplan (Ed.), *Humanscape: Environments for People*. North Situate, MA: Duxubury Press.

Ware, J. (1976). Scales for Measuring General Health Perceptions. *Health Services Research, Winter*, 396-415.

Weinberger, M., Darnel, J., Martz, B., Hiner, S., Neill, P., and Tierney, W. (1986). The Effects of Positive and Negative Life Changes on the Self-Reported Health Status of Elderly Adults. *Journal of Gerontology, 41* (110-114).

Williams, H. (1986). Humor and Healing: Therapeutic Effects in Geriatrics. *Gerontion: A Canadian Review of Geriatric Care, 1*, 14-17.

Young, W. (1982). *The Effect of Humor on Memory*. Washington, DC: Paper presented at the 3rd International Conference on Humor.

Zillmann, L. (1983). Disparagement Humor. In P. McGhee, and J. Goldstein (Ed.), *Handbook of Humor Research*. New York, NY: Springer-Verlag.

Ziv, A. (1982). Cognitive Results of Using Humor in Teaching. Washington, DC: Paper presented at the 3rd International Conference on Humor.

O'Connel, W. (1964). Multidimensional Investigation of Freudian Humor. *Psychi atric Quarterly, 38,* 97-108.

O'Connel, W. (1960). The Adaptive Functions of Wit and Humor. *Journal o Abnormal and Social Psychology, 61,* 263-270.

Paskind, H. (1932). Effects of Laughter on Muscle Tone. *Archives of Neurolog) and Psychiatry, 28* (623-628).

Peter, L., and Dana, B. (1982). *The Laughter Prescription: The Tool of Humor and How to Use it.* New York, NY: Ballantine Books.

Porterfield, A. (1987). Does Sense of Humor Moderate the Impact of Life Stress on Psychological and Physical Well-Being? *Journal of Research in Personality, 21,* 306-317.

Rapp, A. (1951). *The Origin of Wit and Humor.* New York, NY: E. P. Dutton.

Robinson, V. (1970). Humor in Nursing. In C. Carlson, and B. Blackwell (Ed.), *Behavioral Concepts and Nursing Interventions.* Philadelphia, PA: J. B. Lippincott Co.

Robinson, V. (1977). *Humor and the Health Professions.* Thorofore, NJ: Charles B. Slack.

Robinson, V. (1983). Humor and Health. In P. McGhee, and H. Goldstein (Ed.), *Handbook of Humor Research.* New York, NY: Springer-Verlag.

Ryff, C. (1989). In the Eye of the Beholder: Views of Psychological Well-Being Among Middle Aged and Older Adults. *Psychology and Aging, 42*(2), 195-210.

Salameh, W.A. (1983). Humor in Psychotherapy: Past Outlooks, Present Status, and Future Frontiers. In P.E. McGhee and J.H. Goldstein (eds). *Handbook of Humor Research: Volume II Applied Studies.* New York: Springer-Verlag.

Sauer, W. and Warland, R. (1982). Morale and Life Satisfaction. In D. Manger, and W. Peterson (Ed.), *Research Instruments in Social Gerontology.* Minneapolis, MN: University of Minnesota Press.

Schachter, S., and Wheeler, L. (1962). Epinephrine, Chlorpromazine and Amusement. *Journal of Abnormal and Social Psychology, 65* (121-128).

Scheff, T., and Scheele, S. (1979). Humor and Tension: The Effects of Comedy on Audiences. *Catharsis in Healing, Ritual and Drama.* Berkeley, CA: University of California Press.

Schopenhauer, A. (1964). *The World of Will and Ideas.* London, England: Routledge & Kegan Paul.

Schwartz, G. (1974). *Electrographic Studies During Emotions.* Paper presented at the annual meeting of the American Psychosomatic Society.

Simon, J. (1988a). Humor and the Older Adult: Implications for Nursing. *Journal of Advanced Nursing, 13,* 4411-446.

Simon, J. (1988b). The Therapeutic Value of Humor in Aging Adults. *Journal of Gerontological Nursing, 14*(8), 8-13.

Stroufe, L., and Walters, E. (1976). The Ontogenesis of Smiling and Laughter: A Perspective on the Organization of Development in Infancy. *Psychological Review* -83, 173-189.

Sullivan, J., and Deane, D. (1988). Humor and Health. *Journal of Gerontological Nursing,* 14(1), 20-24.